Get Thr

Workpl

Oak Library
The Beeches
Penn Hospital
Wolverhampton

Tel: 01902 695322

Please Return by Last Date Shown Below;

This book is dedicated to:

My beloved wife Dr Mythili Varadan
My beloved sister Mrs Sri Vidhya Rajasekharan
and
To my respected teachers of psychiatry:
  Dr Raja Ram Mohan
  Dr Priscilla Read
  Dr Rhinedd Toms.

Get Through

Workplace Based Assessments in Psychiatry

Second Edition

Sree Prathap Mohana Murthy MB BS MRCPsych

Hertfordshire Partnership NHS Trust

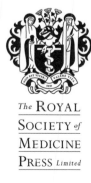

The ROYAL
SOCIETY *of*
MEDICINE
PRESS *Limited*

©2008 Royal Society of Medicine Ltd
Published by the Royal Society of Medicine Press Ltd
1 Wimpole Street, London W1G 0AE, UK
Tel: +44 (0)20 7290 2921
Fax: +44 (0)20 7290 2929
E-mail: publishing@rsmpress.co.uk

British Library Cataloguing in Publication Data
A catalogue record for this book is available from the British Library

ISBN: 978-1-85315-896-4

Distribution in Europe and Rest of the World:
Marston Book Services Ltd
PO Box 269
Abingdon
Oxon OX14 4YN, UK
Tel: +44 (0)1235 465500
Fax: +44 (0)1235 465555
Email: direct.order@marston.co.uk

Distribution in USA and Canada:
Royal Society of Medicine Press Ltd
c/o BookMasters Inc
30 Amberwood Parkway
Ashland, OH 44805, USA
Tel: +1 800 247 6553/ +1 800 266 5564
Fax: +1 410 281 6883
Email: order@bookmasters.com

Distribution in Australia and New Zealand:
Elsevier Australia
30–52 Smidmore Street
Marrickville NSW 2204, Australia
Tel: +61 2 9517 8999
Fax: +61 2 9517 2249
Email: service@elsevier.com.au

Phototypeset by Phoenix Photosetting, Chatham, Kent
Printed in the UK by Bell & Bain Ltd, Glasgow

Contents

Preface

This is one of the first books to be published for helping trainees to perform different workplace based assessments (WPBAs) in psychiatry since this course's implementation by the Royal College of Psychiatrists in August 2007.

This book was initially written to help the candidates to present their long cases in a structured and professional way, however, with the introduction of WPBAs in psychiatry, this book has been revised and is suitable for guidance on how to perform well in all kinds of assessments such as assessed clinical encounters (ACEs), mini-ACEs, case presentations (CPs), case-based discussion (CbD) and direct observation of procedural skills (DOPS).

Get Through Workplace Based Assessments in Psychiatry should be helpful for all the trainees involved in WPBAs in psychiatry – it will not only prepare you to succeed in your WPBAs, but should also help you to face the clinical situations confidently and effectively.

Regards,
Sree Prathap Mohana Murthy

How to use this book

The chapters on eliciting history, mental state examination and physical examination (Chs 2 & 3) could be used for ACEs, mini-ACEs, CbD and CPs in psychiatry. The chapters on differential diagnosis, aetiological formulation, management options and prognosis (Chs 4, 5, 7 & 8) could be used again for ACEs, CPs and CbD on different areas of psychiatry.

I have chosen the individual tasks for mini-ACEs from different areas of psychiatry, which could be applied to a wide variety of settings. I have also included some tasks for DOPS in psychiatry.

General management options are also discussed (with evidence and key points) for all the common psychiatric conditions seen in our routine practice, including subspecialties such as old age psychiatry, child and adolescent psychiatry and learning disability.

You can quickly revise the management plans before presenting the case to the assessor, and you may find it helpful to establish a confident discussion with the assessors as part of your assessment.

The answers that I have given should only be used as a rough guide, and reference to standard textbooks is also recommended.

In short, this book could be used as a 'pocket revision guide' for all trainees in psychiatry involved in WPBAs, which constitutes a significant part of their current training.

I sincerely hope that this book serves its purpose! Good luck.

SPMM

1

Introduction to workplace based assessments (WPBAs)

The Royal College curriculum for specialist training in psychiatry is supported by an extensive assessment programme comprising both workplace based assessments and formal MRCPsych examinations.

Key methods and instruments of WPBA would include:

1. Assessment of clinical expertise (ACE)
2. Mini-assessed clinical encounter (mini-ACE)
3. Case based discussion (CbD)
4. Case presentation (CP)
5. Directly observed procedural skills (DOPS)
6. Journal club presentation (JCP)
7. Mini-peer assessment tool (mini-PAT)

This book is mainly intended to be used for the *first five WPBAs listed above.*

The underlying principles of WPBAs must comply with the following (Royal College, 2007):

● They must focus on performance
● They must be evidence-based
● The evidence must be triangulated whenever possible
● Record must be permanent.

According to the Royal College guidelines, participating in a specific number of WPBAs is mandatory for eligibility for the MRCPsych examinations.

All the WPBA forms use a six-point Likert-type rating scale. The standard for completion of each stage of training corresponds to a rating of 4. Most assessment forms would also have an additional item to indicate the trainee's global performance relative to their stage of training. These forms are available to download from http://www.rcpsych.ac.uk/wba.

The assessments should be followed by immediate feedback to the trainee, which would involve going through the rating form item by item, so that strengths, weaknesses and areas for development can be identified and agreed.

Assessor: Consultant, specialist registrar, associate specialist, senior nurse, psychologist, social worker. (A variety of different assessors can be used.)

TABLE 1.1 Annual requirements for work place based assessments

WPBA	Minimum number required per year
ACE	2 in ST1
	3 in ST2
	3 in ST3
Mini-ACE	4
CbD	2
CP	1
DOPS	As the opportunity arises
JCP	1
Mini-PAT	2
AoT	As the opportunity arises

Assessment of clinical expertise (ACE)

The ACE component of WPBA most closely resembles the traditional long case assessment. Here the assessor observes a whole new patient encounter to assess your ability to take both a full comprehensive history and mental state examination, arrive at a diagnosis and formulate a management plan.

The Assessor rates the performance, and then gives immediate feedback to the trainee and the assessment takes about an hour to complete, including the time taken by the assessor to complete the ACE rating form.

The domains of assessment would include:

- History taking
- Mental state examination
- Communication skills
- Clinical judgement
- Professionalism
- Organizational efficiency
- Overall clinical care.

Mini-assessed clinical encounter (mini-ACE)

The mini-ACE could be used for short focused tasks, to elicit key important elements from the history or mental state. Rather than taking a full history and performing a complete examination, the focus is on clearly defined clinical competencies, and the trainee is asked to conduct a focused interview and examination, for example, alcohol history taking, assessment of a cognitive state, suicide risk assessment.

It is a snapshot of a clinical interaction between doctor and patient with the assessor observing only part of a patient interaction. The mini-ACE is considered to have similarities with the 'observed interview' part of the traditional long case examination of the MRCPsych.

The assessor rates the performance, and then gives immediate feedback to the trainee and the assessment takes about 20 minutes, followed by 5–10 minutes of feedback (approximately 30 minutes in total).

Different assessors would assess each trainee on several different occasions over a range of clinical settings such as inpatient, outpatient, community and A&E.

The domains of assessment would be the same as those of the ACEs, with the only difference here being that the trainee is rated in the context of a 'shorter clinical assessment':

- History taking
- Mental state examination
- Communication skills
- Clinical judgement
- Professionalism
- Organizational efficiency
- Overall clinical care.

Case-based discussion (CbD)

The CbD component of WPBA involves the trainee selecting two case records of patients seen, in whose notes they have made an entry, and the assessor picks one to discuss, e.g., a patient with bipolar disorder assessed during a home visit).

It allows the assessor to examine different areas such as clinical decision-making, the application of medical knowledge, and discussion of the ethical and legal framework, with the discussion originating from the entries made in the clinical notes by trainees. It also provides an opportunity for the trainee to explain the decision and justify their actions taken.

The process is trainee-led and takes about 15–20 minutes, followed by 5–10 minutes' feedback (approximately 30 minutes in total).

It enables an assessor to provide systematic assessment and structured feedback to the trainee.

The domains of assessment would include:

- Clinical record keeping
- Clinical assessment including diagnostic skills

- Risk assessment and management
- Medical treatment
- Investigation and referral
- Follow-up and care planning
- Professionalism
- Clinical reasoning (includes decision making skills)
- Overall clinical care.

Case presentation (CP)

The case presentation assessment assesses the trainee's participation in the overall clinical management of the patient as well as their presentation skills.

The domains of assessment would include:

- Assessment and clinical examination
- Interpretation of clinical evidence
- Use of investigations
- Presentation and delivery
- Global rating.

There should be at least 5 minutes of feedback from the assessor at the completion of the presentation.

ST4, ST5 and ST6 continue this development, extending into the trainee's specialist areas of psychiatry. It is also an attempt to assess activities such as grand rounds in a structured way as part of competency assessment.

Direct observation of procedural skills (DOPS)

Although DOPS has more limited use in psychiatry compared with other areas of medicine, it can be used in situations such as administering electroconvulsive therapy (ECT) or conducting a risk assessment in a patient who has recently taken an overdose. It not only assesses practical skills but also assesses important communication skills.

The assessment should normally take 10–15 minutes with the assessor giving immediate feedback to the trainee, which takes about 5 minutes.

The domains of assessment would include:

- Understanding of indications, relevant anatomy, technique of procedure
- Obtaining informed consent
- Appropriate pre-procedure preparation
- Appropriate analgesia or safe sedation
- Technical ability

- Aseptic technique
- Seeking help where appropriate
- Post-procedure management
- Communication skills
- Consideration of patient/professionalism
- Overall ability to perform procedure.

> DOPS: 'Its application in psychiatry will be further developed and it also might be necessary to modify the assessment form to make it more widely applicable to psychiatry and it might also be necessary to define "procedures" relevant to the speciality of psychiatry more carefully to avoid significant overlap in the purpose of the various assessment tools.'
>
> (Bhugra et al, 2007)

2

History taking and mental state examination

How to take a history

- The history taking should begin with a courteous introduction and explanation of the interview, and any patient questions and concerns should be addressed first.
- Don't be hurried; act naturally, and be genuine, polite and professional with the patient.
- Be respectful and empathetic with the patient.
- Do not disagree with improbable assertions, such as delusional ideas or other psychotic phenomena, but avoid debating them.
- Do not focus too much on irrelevances, but try to redirect the flow of conversation and tailor the interview accordingly.
- Keep safety issues in mind throughout the assessment.
- The closure of the interview should be generally supportive and should include thanking the patient and providing an opportunity for the patient to ask questions or add any other information that is significant to the case.
- There are different schools of thought regarding the subheadings of a history, but the following format is usually accepted by most assessors/trainers:
  - Demographic details
  - Reason for referral
  - Chief complaints
  - History of presenting complaints
  - Past psychiatric history
  - Past medical history
  - Current medications
  - Family history
  - Personal history
  - Current social circumstances (social history)
  - Drug and alcohol history
  - Forensic history

- Premorbid personality
- Mental state examination.

Demographic data

- Name
- Age
- Sex
- Marital status
- Employment status
- Occupation
- Date of admission (if applicable)
- Legal status (if applicable).

Reason for referral

- How did you come into the hospital?
- Who referred you?
- When were you referred?
- Why were you referred?
- Did you come of your own free will or were you forced to come?

Chief complaints

Establish exactly why the patient came to see the psychiatrist, preferably using the patient's own words.

- What are your main problems or your main concerns?
- Specifically try to identify:
    - What is the nature of the problem?
    - Why and how has the individual presented this time?
    - What events led up to this presentation?

History of presenting complaints

- Identify specific symptoms that are present and their duration:
    - *Chronological order:* Which symptom started first?
    - *Onset and duration:* How did it start? Was it slowly, gradually, rapidly or suddenly? When did you last feel well?
    - *Course:* Did it get better, worse, remain the same, or was it up and down?

- Impairment in *normal functioning* (domestic, social and occupational functioning) – the impact of symptoms on patient, family, work and social life:
  - I would like to know how your problems have been affecting you, your family and your social life.
  - How does it interfere with your normal life and activities?
- *Recent stressors*/stressful life events: note the time relationship between the onset of the current symptoms and the presence of social stressors/ stressful life events.
- Disturbance in *biological* symptoms:
  - Sleep
  - Appetite
  - Libido
  - Weight.
- Also obtain information about any treatments for the problem and the individual's response to treatment.

Screening questions: direct questioning

Start with open questions and then proceed to closed questions; and screen them for different types of symptoms. (The questions to be asked under each category are discussed in detail in Chapter 9.)

Past psychiatric history

- Have you ever had problems with your mental health/nerves/depression?
- Have you ever seen a psychiatrist before?
- Have you ever been admitted to a psychiatric hospital?
  - If so, ask about previous psychiatric episodes – the symptoms, complaints, precipitants, where they were seen, by whom and the diagnosis, if known.
- What treatments have you had before and what was the response?
  - Type of treatment – inpatient/outpatient, informal/detention.
- Has there ever been a time when you felt completely well?
- Also ask about inter-episode functioning (psychiatric state between episodes – whether completely well or maintained on treatment).
- Have you ever attempted to harm yourself in the past? History of overdoses, deliberate self harm (DSH) or attempted suicide.

Past medical history

- Do you have any problems with your physical health?
- What about in the past? Any medical illnesses?
- Have you ever had any operations or been in the hospital?
- Have you ever had any accidents, head injury or loss of consciousness?

Current medications

- What medications do you take regularly?
- What medications have you had in the past?
- Are you allergic to any medications?

Family history

'Now, I would like to ask you a few questions about yourself and your background.'

Enquire about parents, siblings, grandparents, cousins, and adoptive/foster/step-parents:

- Tell me about your parents. Your mum and dad ...
  - How old are they?
  - What did your parents work at?
  - How did you get along with your parents?
  - How did your parents get along together?
- Do you have any brothers or sisters? Tell me about them.
- As far as you know, has anyone in your family or blood relatives ever had problems with their mental health?

Also, ask for history of suicides/alcoholism/epilepsy in the family.

Personal history

'I would like to talk now about your childhood, education and adolescence.'

Childhood

- Where were you born?
- Where were you brought up? And by whom?
- As far as you know was your mother's pregnancy normal?
- Was it a normal delivery?

- Were there any problems around the time of your birth or when you were growing up?
- Were you walking and talking at the correct times?
- Did you have any serious illness as a young child?
- When did you start school, and when did you finish school?
- Which schools did you go to?
- Did you enjoy school?
- Did you have any problems at school?
- Did you have many friends at school?
- Have you ever been bullied or did you bully others?
- Did you play truant? Were you ever expelled or suspended from school?
- When did you leave school?
- Did you gain any qualification at school?
- What did you do after finishing school? Did you go to college or university?
- Ask about college (subjects and qualifications) and other post-school training.
- How would you describe your childhood?
- Ask in particular about:
  - Any major loss during childhood
  - Separations
  - Childhood neglect
  - Physical/emotional/sexual abuses in childhood
  - Sibling rivalry.

Work history

Enquire about the jobs held, nature of work, reasons for leaving jobs and any periods of unemployment.

- What did you work at? For how long? Then what happened?
- How many steady jobs did you have?
- What is your current job? How do you feel about your current job? Any problems with the job/colleagues?
- Are you unemployed at the moment? If so, why?

Psychosexual history

- Tell me about your partner/wife.
- How long have you been with your current partner?
- Are you married at present?
- How would you describe your marriage?
- How do you get on with her?
- Have you had any difficulties in your current relationship?
- Do you have children? If so, how many, and how old are they?

- How is your relationship with your children?
- How many previous relationships have you had?
- Tell me more about your previous relationships, previous partners/separations/divorces?

Current social circumstances

Social support

- Who lives at home with you at the moment?
- Do you have friends or family who live nearby?

Housing

Type of accommodation:
- – Own/rented/council?
- – Flat/house/bungalow?

How long have you been living there?

Finances and employment

- Employed/unemployed? Where do you work?
- What is your source of income?
- Enquire about income support/disability living allowance/state pension.
- Do you have any worries about debt or money in general?

Other support

Also enquire about other support such as community psychiatric nurse input, social workers' input, carer input, support workers and voluntary agencies.

Drug and alcohol history

Enquire about smoking, alcohol and illicit drugs. If there is any positive history, explore further.

Smoking history

- Do you smoke?
- How much and how often in a day?
- Tell me more about it.

Alcohol history

- Do you drink alcohol?
- What do you usually drink?
- How often do you have a drink?
- How many drinks do you have on a typical day of drinking?
- What type of effect does alcohol have on you?
- How much money do you spend per day/week on drinking alcohol?
- When did it all start?
- How did you progress to the current level?
- Ask about details of treatment and details of any period of abstinence or binge drinking.
- Any detoxification programme? Was it completed?

Illicit drug history

- Have you ever used any recreational drugs such as cannabis, cocaine/crack, amphetamines, speed, ecstasy, LSD (or) acid? Ask about individual drugs by naming them.
- What drugs are you using now?
- Tell me more about it.
- How often do you take these drugs?
- What is the amount of drug taken?
- How much money do you spend in a day/week to get these drugs?
- What is the route of use – oral, smoked, snorted, injected? If drugs are injected, the following questions are useful:
    - Are needles used?
    - Where are they obtained?
    - Are needles shared?
    - What sites are used for injection?
- What effect is the patient seeking when using the drug?
- Ask whether more than one drug is used at a time.
- How is the patient financing the drug use?

For more questions please see *Eliciting alcohol history and illicit drug history* in Chapter 9.

Forensic history

- Have you ever been in trouble with the police or broken the law?
- Have you ever been charged or convicted of anything?
- Have you ever been involved with any criminal activity?
- If any, what are the offences/crimes that you have committed?

- Have you served any period in prison/probation/on remand?

Try to obtain a list of offences, charges, legal outcome and length and place of any prison sentence.

Premorbid personality

Start with open questions:

- How would you describe yourself as a person before you were ill?
- How do you think other people would describe you as a person?

Then ask closed questions about individual personality traits:

- Predominant mood:
  - Optimistic/pessimistic
  - Stable/prone to anxiety
  - Cheerful/despondent
- Interpersonal relationships:
  - Current friendships and relationships, previous relationships – ability to establish and maintain
  - Family relationships
- Coping strategies:
  - When you find yourself in difficult situations, what do you do to cope?
  - What sort of things do you like to do to relax?
- Personal interests:
  - Hobbies and interests
  - Use of leisure time
- Beliefs – religious beliefs
- Habits – food, fads, etc.

Cluster A, Cluster B, Cluster C personality types – for more questions please see *Eliciting premorbid personality*, Chapter 9.

> 'History taking is never a completed task, no matter how long you have known the patient. No one can ever know everything about another human being.'
>
> Rob Poole and Robert Higgo

Mental state examination

Appearance and behaviour

- Apparent age, stature, race
- Dressed, kempt, groomed
- Self-neglecting features

- Eye contact and rapport
- Posture, facial expression, mannerisms
- Prominent physical characteristics – scars, tattoos, etc.
- Psychomotor changes, voluntary and involuntary movements, catatonic features.

Speech

- Rate
- Tone and volume
- Relevancy and coherency.

Mood

- Subjective mood – predominant mood in patient's own words.
- Objective mood – euthymic/euphoric/dysthymic/dysphoric, apprehensive/angry/apathetic (your appraisal).

Affect

- Labile, flat, blunt, reactive, congruent/incongruent.

Thought

- Thought processes:
  - Logical, coherent and goal-directed
  - Loosening of association/blocking/perseveration
  - Tangentiality/circumstantiality/neologisms
- Thought content – mention only positive findings:
  - Predominant topic or issue, preoccupations, ruminations
  - Unusual ideas or concerns
  - Obsessions, phobias and overvalued ideas
  - Ask specifically for suicidal and/or homicidal ideation – suicidal ideas/intentions/plans
  - Feelings of hopelessness or helplessness, ideas of worthlessness
- Abnormal beliefs:
  - Delusions – content of any delusional system, its organization, the patient's convictions as to its validity and the type of delusions
  - Passivity phenomena.

Perception

- Illusions
- Hallucinations

- Depersonalization
- Derealization.

Cognition

Give a brief summary when all aspects of the cognitive state are normal; or a more detailed summary when some aspects are abnormal but not clinically decisive; or a full summary of testing when the results are diagnostically significant.

Orientation

- Time (day, date, year, time of the day)
- Place (name of the place/hospital/floor)
- Person.

Attention and concentration

- Subtracting a series of 7s from 100
- Days of the week forwards/backwards
- Months of the year forwards/backwards.

Memory

Working memory – digit span 6 plus or minus 1

Short-term memory – name and address: immediate and delayed (5-minute recall)

Long-term memory:

Personal events:
a. When did you get married?
b. When did you finish school?
General events:
a. Who is the current prime minister of the UK?
b. Who is the current president of the USA?
c. What are the years of World War II?

Insight

- Recognition and attribution of illness
- Awareness of treatment that includes benefits of having the treatment and adherence/compliance to treatment.

3

Physical examination

Try to look for relevant findings related to the psychiatric and medical history.

Aims of routine physical examination

- To assess the patient's baseline physical state
- To identify the presence or absence of any abnormal signs that could be associated with their physical or mental health condition
- To identify areas that require further examination, investigation and treatment.

General examination

- Height and weight
- Bruises, scars, tattoos
- Any evidence of previous injury (e.g., self-cutting, etc.)
- Any signs of recent weight loss
- Any signs of physical neglect
- Vital signs:
  - Heart rate
  - Blood pressure
  - Respiratory rate
  - Temperature
  - Evidence of autonomic arousal, such as sweating, tremor or pallor.

Specific system examinations

These are to be done briefly. It is very important to examine what the history indicates is pertinent.

The specific system examination should focus on the following:

- Cardiovascular examination
  - Blood pressure
  - Radial pulse-rate, rhythm and character
  - Heart sounds
  - Carotid bruits
  - Pedal oedema.
- Respiratory examination
  - Respiratory rate
  - Chest expansion
  - Percussion note
  - Auscultatory breath sounds
- Gastrointestinal examination
  - Any swelling, ascites or palpable masses
  - Bowel sounds
  - Hernias
- Central nervous system examination – full neurological examination is the most important of all
  - Examination of all four limbs for tone, power, reflexes, weakness and altered sensation
  - Gait inspection
  - Examination of hand–eye coordination
  - Check for involuntary movements
  - Cranial nerve examination
  - Fundoscopy (only if necessary)
- Stigmata of liver disease – jaundice, spider naevi, gynaecomastia, palmar erythema, hepatomegaly
- Stigmata of thyroid disease:
  - Hyperthyroidism – agitation, sweating, tremor, exophthalmos, lid-lag, pretibial myxoedema, thyroid bruit
  - Hypothyroidism – dry scaly skin, dry brittle hair, hair loss, goitre, hoarse voice, weight gain, sinus bradycardia, slow-relaxing reflexes, psycho-motor retardation
- Look for features of alcohol/drug intoxication and withdrawal features:
  - Features of alcohol withdrawal – sweating, tremor, tachycardia, nausea, vomiting, generalized anxiety, psychomotor agitation, occasional visual, tactile or auditory hallucination
  - Features of opiate withdrawal – watering eyes and nose, yawning, nausea, vomiting, diarrhoea, tremor, joint pains, muscle cramps,

sweating, dilated pupils, tachycardia, hypertension, piloerection (goose-flesh)
- Look for features of extrapyramidal signs such as akathisia, dystonias, tremor, rigidity and dyskinesias
- Any other finding that is clearly relevant for your case – for example, in a patient with significant history of alcohol abuse, look for:
  - Signs of alcohol withdrawal (tremor at rest, tachycardia, perspiration)
  - Signs of liver disease (jaundice, spider naevi, palmar erythema, hepatomegaly)
  - Neurological signs (ataxia, nystagmus, dysarthria and peripheral neuropathy).

Summary

Summary of positive findings and significant information relevant to the case obtained from history, mental state examination and physical examination.

4

Diagnosis and differential diagnoses

Diagnosis

All diagnostic features described below are based mainly on ICD-10 criteria.

Schizophrenia

A diagnosis of schizophrenia can be made if there is one clear symptom, or usually two or more symptoms if less clear-cut, which should have been clearly present for most of the time during a period of 1 month or more.

At least *one* of the following:

- Delusions of thought interference (thought withdrawal, thought insertion, thought broadcasting) or thought echo
- Delusions of control, influence or passivity; delusional perception
- Running commentary hallucinations; third-person hallucinations; hallucinations from part of the body
- Bizarre persistent delusions of other kinds that are culturally inappropriate and completely impossible.

A diagnosis of schizophrenia can also be made if symptoms from at least two of the groups listed below have been clearly present for most of the time during a period of *1 month or more*.

At least *two* of the following:

- Persistent hallucinations in any modality when accompanied by fleeting or half-formed delusions
- Breaks or interpolations in the train of thought leading to irrelevant, incoherent speech or neologisms
- Catatonic symptoms
- Negative symptoms
- A significant and consistent change in the overall quality of some aspects of the patient's behaviour.

If the symptoms are present for a duration of less than 1 month, it should be diagnosed in the first instance as acute schizophrenia-like psychotic disorder and should later be reclassified as schizophrenia if the symptoms persist for longer periods.

Paranoid schizophrenia

The general criteria for a diagnosis of schizophrenia must be satisfied. The clinical picture is often characterized by paranoid delusions (delusions of persecution, delusions of reference, control, passivity) usually accompanied by auditory hallucinations, other perceptual disturbances and hallucinations of the other modalities. In addition, disturbances of affect, volition, and speech may also be present.

Schizoaffective disorder

Schizoaffective disorder is characterized by having affective and schizophrenic symptoms, both prominent within the same episode of illness simultaneously or within a few days of each other, and they should be equally prominent.

It excludes patients with separate episodes of schizophrenia and affective disorders.

Mood-incongruent delusions or hallucinations in affective disorders do not justify a diagnosis of schizoaffective disorder.

Schizoaffective disorder, manic type

In this disorder, schizophrenic symptoms and manic symptoms are both prominent in the same episode of illness. There must be a prominent elevation of mood, and at least one, and preferably two, schizophrenic symptoms as specified for schizophrenia should be clearly present.

Schizoaffective disorder, depressive type

In this disorder, schizophrenic symptoms and depressive symptoms are both prominent in the same episode of illness. There must be prominent depressive symptoms accompanied by at least two characteristic symptoms, and also at least one, or preferably two, schizophrenic symptoms as specified for schizophrenia should be clearly present.

Schizoaffective disorder, mixed type

Here, symptoms of schizophrenia coexist with those of a mixed bipolar affective disorder.

Persistent delusional disorder

- Circumscribed symptoms of non-bizarre delusions
- Absence of prominent hallucinations
- No evidence of thought disorder or mood disorder
- Symptoms should have been present for at least 3 months.

Depression

Typical symptoms:

- Depressed mood
- Anhedonia (loss of interest and enjoyment)
- Reduced energy leading to increased fatiguability and diminished activity.

Core symptoms:

- Poor memory, reduced attention and concentration
- Low self-esteem, reduced self confidence
- Ideas of guilt, bleak and pessimistic views of the future, unworthiness
- Ideas or acts of self-harm or suicide
- Disturbed sleep
- Diminished appetite.

Classification:

- Mild depressive episode – at least two of the typical symptoms plus at least two of the core symptoms
- Moderate depressive episode – at least two of the typical symptoms should be present plus at least three, and preferably four, of the core symptoms
- Severe depressive episode – all three of the typical symptoms should be present plus at least four of the core symptoms, some of which should be of severe intensity.

Step 1: Decide if mild, moderate or severe and also assess the degree of functional impairment

For depressive episodes, a duration of at least 2 weeks is usually required for diagnosis, but if the symptoms are particularly severe and of very rapid onset, it may be justified to make this diagnosis after less than 2 weeks.

The differentiation between the three grades rests upon a complicated clinical judgement that involves the number, type and severity of symptoms present plus the extent of impairment in social and work activities.

Step 2: Somatic syndrome present/absent

Somatic symptoms:

- Loss of interest or pleasure in activities that are usually enjoyable
- Early morning awakening – at least 2 hours before the usual time
- Diurnal variation of mood, being worst in the morning
- Weight loss (5% or more of body weight in the last month)
- Marked loss of appetite
- Marked loss of libido
- Objective evidence of definite psychomotor retardation or agitation.

With somatic syndrome, four or more of the somatic symptoms should be present.

The use of this category may be justified if only two or three somatic symptoms are present, but they are unusually severe.

It is presumed that the somatic syndrome will almost always be present in a severe depressive episode.

Step 3: Psychotic symptoms present/absent

Psychotic symptoms involve a severe depressive episode in which delusions, hallucinations or depressive stupor are present and the delusions or hallucinations may be specified as mood congruent or mood incongruent.

Step 4: Assess suicidality

Assess suicidality of a patient presenting with low mood.

Recurrent depressive disorder

The disorder is characterized by repeated episodes of depression without any history of independent episodes of mood elevation and overactivity that fulfil the criteria of mania.

It occurs in the following forms:

- Recurrent depressive disorder, current episode mild, with/without somatic syndrome
- Recurrent depressive disorder, current episode moderate, with/without somatic syndrome
- Recurrent depressive disorder, current episode severe without psychotic symptoms
- Recurrent depressive disorder, current episode severe with psychotic symptoms.

Mania

Decide if it is hypomania or mania with/without psychotic symptoms.

Hypomania

- Persistent mild elation of mood (for at least several days on end)
- Increased energy and activity
- Marked feelings of well-being, both physical and mental efficiency
- Over familiarity, talkativeness, increased sociability
- Increased sexual energy and decreased need for sleep
- Impaired attention and concentration
- Mild overspending and development of new interests.

In hypomania, the symptoms are often present but not to the extent that they lead to severe disruption of work or social functioning.

Mania (without psychotic symptoms)

- Elevated mood (not in keeping with the individual's circumstance)
- Increased energy resulting in overactivity
- Disinhibition, excessive spending
- Accelerated thoughts and pressure of speech
- Decreased need for sleep, appetite disturbance, increased libido
- Distractibility, impaired attention and concentration
- Inflated self-esteem and grandiose or freely expressed overoptimistic ideas.

The episode should last for 1 week and should be severe enough to disrupt social or occupational life more or less completely.

Mania (with psychotic symptoms)

- The clinical picture is that of a more severe form of mania
- Delusions – delusions of persecution, delusions of grandiosity, religious delusions
- Delusions or hallucinations can be specified as mood congruent or mood incongruent.

Bipolar affective disorder

Bipolar affective disorder is characterized by repeated episodes (at least two) of hypomania/mania and depression, and the recovery is complete between the episodes.

Bipolar affective disorder, hypomania

The present episode should fulfil the criteria for hypomania, and there must have been at least one other affective episode in the past (hypomania, mania, depression or mixed).

Bipolar affective disorder, manic without psychotic symptoms

The present episode should fulfil the criteria for mania without psychotic symptoms, and there must have been at least one other affective episode in the past (hypomania, mania, depression or mixed).

Bipolar affective disorder, manic with psychotic symptoms

The present episode should fulfil the criteria for mania with psychotic symptoms, and there must have been at least one other affective episode in the past (hypomania, mania, depression or mixed).

Bipolar affective disorder, current episode mild or moderate depression

The present episode should fulfil the criteria for a depressive episode of either mild or moderate severity, and there must have been at least one other affective episode in the past (hypomania, mania, depression or mixed).

Bipolar affective disorder, current episode severe depression without psychotic symptoms

The present episode should fulfil the criteria for a severe depressive episode without psychotic symptoms, and there must have been at least one other affective episode in the past (hypomania, mania, depression or mixed).

Bipolar affective disorder, current episode severe depression with psychotic symptoms

The present episode should fulfil the criteria for a severe depressive episode with psychotic symptoms, and there must have been at least one other affective episode in the past (hypomania, mania, depression or mixed).

Bipolar affective disorder, current episode mixed

The patient has had at least one hypomania, manic or mixed affective episode in the past and currently exhibits both manic and depressive symptoms, both prominent for the greater part of the current episode, and the episode must have lasted for at least 2 weeks.

Generalized anxiety disorder

At least *four* of the following types of symptom should be present, and the symptoms should be present most days for at least 6 months:

- Autonomic arousal: palpitations, tachycardia, sweating, dry mouth, trembling and shaking
- Physical symptoms: difficulty in breathing, chest pain/discomfort, choking sensation, nausea and abdominal distress, difficulty swallowing
- Mental state symptoms: dizziness, light-headedness, fear of losing control, fear of dying or fear of 'going crazy'
- General symptoms: numbness, tingling sensations, hot flushes
- Symptoms of tension: muscular tension, aches and pains, feeling 'on the edge', inability to relax
- Others: exaggerated startle response, persistent irritability, concentration difficulties, difficulty getting to sleep.

Agoraphobia with (or without) panic disorder

Diagnosis in ICD-10:

- Symptoms of anxiety (including psychological, behavioural and autonomic symptoms) should be present, and they are not secondary to other symptoms, delusions or obsessions.
- Anxiety occurs in at least two of the following situations: crowds, public places, travelling alone, travelling away from home.
- Avoidance behaviour: avoidance of the phobic situation as a prominent feature.

Social phobia

- Symptoms of anxiety (including psychological, behavioural and autonomic symptoms) should be present, and they are not secondary to other symptoms, delusions or obsessions.
- Anxiety occurs particularly in social situations (restricted to eating in public, public speaking, encounters with the opposite sex).
- Avoidance behaviour: avoidance of the phobic situation as a prominent feature. There may be associated blushing, nausea and hand tremor, often leading to avoidance behaviour and alcohol misuse.

Specific phobia

- Symptoms of anxiety (including psychological, behavioural and autonomic symptoms) should be present, and they are not secondary to other symptoms, delusions or obsessions.

- The anxiety must be restricted to the presence of the particular phobic object or situation.
- Avoidance behaviour: avoidance of the phobic situation as a prominent feature. There may be associated blushing, nausea and hand tremor, often leading to avoidance behaviour and alcohol misuse.

Panic disorder (episodic paroxysmal anxiety)

Essential features are recurrent; unpredictable attacks of panic in a range of situations.
Diagnosis in ICD-10:

- Several severe attacks within the last month:
  - In circumstances where there is no objective danger
  - Not confined to known or predictable situations
- Freedom from anxiety symptoms between attacks.

Obsessive–compulsive disorder

Symptoms (obsessional symptoms or compulsive acts) must be present on most days over the preceding 2 weeks, causing distress and interference with normal activities.

- Recognized as the individual's own thoughts or impulses
- Resistance: there must be at least one thought or act that is still resisted unsuccessfully
- Ritual is not in itself pleasurable
- Thoughts, images or impulses must be unpleasantly repetitive.

Post-traumatic stress disorder

- Extreme nature of traumatic event
- Onset follows the trauma with a latency period that may range from a few weeks to months, but rarely exceeds 6 months
- Symptoms of increased psychological sensitivity and arousal: difficulty in concentration, irritability, sleep disturbances, exaggerated startle response and hypervigilance
- Persistent reliving of the event in recurring dreams, nightmares, vivid memories and flashbacks
- Avoidance: actual or preferred avoidance of situations/circumstances associated with the stressor, which are a reminder of the event
- General lack of interest, detachment and numbness.

Adjustment disorder

- Onset within 1 month of stressful event or life change
- Duration of symptoms does not usually exceed 6 months
- States of subjective distress and emotional disturbance, usually interfering with normal social functioning and performance, and arising in the period of adaptation to a significant life change or to the consequences of a stressful life event (including the presence or possibility of serious physical illness).

Anorexia nervosa

- Weight loss >15% of total body weight and below-expected body mass index (BMI) of 17.5 or less
- Body image distortion – fear of fatness held as an overvalued idea
- Avoidance of fattening foods, with behaviours aimed at losing weight, such as vomiting, purging, over-exercise and use of appetite suppressants
- Amenorrhoea, reduced sexual interest, impotence
- Pubertal delay if onset is early.

Bulimia nervosa

- Persistent preoccupation with and irresistible craving for food
- Binges – episodes of overeating
- Avoidance of fattening foods, with behaviours aimed at losing weight such as vomiting, purging, over-exercise and use of appetite suppressants
- Morbid fear of fatness with imposed 'low weight threshold'.

Alcohol/drug dependence syndrome

Edwards and Gross criteria (1976):

- Loss of control of consumption
- Increased tolerance to the effects of drugs
- Signs of withdrawal on attempted abstinence
- Relief of withdrawal symptoms by drinking or by taking drugs
- Rapid reinstatement of previous pattern of drug use after abstinence
- Continued use despite negative consequences
- Narrowing of the drinking/drug-taking repertoire
- Primacy of drug-seeking behaviour.

Emotionally unstable personality disorder

Borderline type

- Boredom and chronic emptiness
- Identity confusion

- Recurrent suicide threats or acts of self-harm
- Impulsivity
- Relationship difficulties – intense and unstable relationships
- Affective instability – unpredictable affect.

Impulsive type

- Inability to control anger
- Unpredictable affect and behaviour.

Dementia in Alzheimer's disease

- Global deterioration in intellectual capacity and disturbance in higher cortical functions, such as memory, thinking, orientation, comprehension, calculation, language, learning abilities and judgement; an appreciable decline in intellectual functioning and some interference with personal activities of daily living
- Insidious onset with slow deterioration
- Absence of clinical evidence or findings from special investigations suggestive of organic brain disease or other systemic abnormalities
- Absence of sudden onset or physical/neurological signs.

Remember 5 As

- Amnesia – impaired ability to learn new information and to recall previously learned information
- Aphasia – problems with language (receptive and expressive)
- Agnosia – failure of recognition, especially people
- Apraxia – inability to carry out purposeful movements even though there is no sensory or motor impairment
- Associated disturbance – behavioural changes, delusions, hallucinations.

Vascular dementia

- Presence of a dementia syndrome, defined by cognitive decline from a previously higher level of functioning and manifested by impairment of memory and of two or more cognitive domains (orientation, attention, language, visuospatial functions, executive functions, motor control and praxis), and deficits should be severe enough to interfere with activities of daily living not due to physical effects of stroke alone
- Onset may be gradual as in some subtypes, or it can be abrupt following one particular ischaemic episode
- Course is usually stepwise, with periods of intervening stability

- Focal neurological signs and symptoms or neurological evidence of cerebrovascular disease (CVD) judged aetiologically related to the disturbance. CVD defined by the presence of focal signs on neurological examination, such as hemiparesis, lower facial weakness, Babinski sign, sensory deficit, hemianopia and dysarthria and evidence of relevant CVD by brain imaging (CT or MRI)
- Relative preservation of personality and insight
- Emotional and personality changes are typically early, followed by cognitive deficits that are often fluctuating in severity
- Symptoms not occurring during the course of the delirium.

Lewy body dementia

- Fluctuating cognitive impairment affecting both memory and higher cortical functions; fluctuation is pronounced with both episodic confusion and lucid intervals as in delirium
- Prominent visual hallucinations and/or auditory hallucinations usually accompanied by secondary paranoid delusions; the whole spectrum of psychiatric presentations can also occur
- Motor features of parkinsonism
- Neuroleptic sensitivity – exaggerated form of response to standard doses of neuroleptics
- Repeated unexplained falls.

Note: If both motor and cognitive symptoms develop within 12 months, it is conventional to give a diagnosis of Lewy body dementia. A diagnosis of *Parkinson's disease dementia* is given if the parkinsonian symptoms have existed for at least 12 months before dementia develops and the dementing process develops in the course of established Parkinson's disease.

Frontotemporal dementia

- Insidious onset and gradual progression
- Early loss of personal and social awareness
- Early emotional blunting; early loss of insight
- Behavioural features: early signs of disinhibition, decline in personal hygiene and grooming, mental rigidity, inflexibility, hyperorality, stereotyped and perseverative behaviour
- Speech disorder: reduction and stereotypy of speech, echolalia, and perseveration
- Affective symptoms: anxiety, depression, and frequent mood changes, emotional indifference
- Physical signs: incontinence, primitive reflexes, akinesia, rigidity and tremor.

Differential diagnosis

Work out the differential diagnosis by applying the diagnostic hierarchy and process of exclusion.

- Organic illness, epilepsy, drug- and alcohol-induced illness
- Schizophrenia and other psychotic disorders
- Affective disorders
- Neurotic disorders, eating disorders, post-traumatic stress disorder (PTSD), somatization disorders
- Personality traits/disorders.

Useful hints

- Know the ICD-10 well as it is the basis for differential diagnosis. You should, therefore, familiarize yourself with this classification, and it can be very helpful to have pre-prepared a list of standardized differential diagnoses for the common presenting problems that we come across in our day-to-day practice.
- Proceed as follows:
  - Prepare a list of all the diagnoses you wish to present.
  - Give the reasons for and against each diagnosis.
  - Make clear which are competing diagnoses (i.e. the main differentials) and which are additional diagnoses, e.g., severe depression with psychotic symptoms, with a number of competing diagnostic possibilities as well as alcohol dependence and a dependent personality.
  - Also make clear if you consider one (or more than one) diagnosis is clearly preferable.
  - Carefully review organic possibilities (such as withdrawal from substance misuse) and include them wherever there is some clinical indication.
  - Only state actual possibilities, and, if you are really considering them in the differential for your particular case, be prepared to justify your reasons.

Here below, I have discussed in detail the differential diagnoses of common psychiatric conditions that we come across in our clinical practice.

Schizophrenia

- Organic psychotic disorder:
  - Drug-induced psychosis; related to substance misuse, drug intoxication and withdrawal with stimulants (cannabis, cocaine, LSD, amphetamine and ecstasy)

- Delirium
- Related to a general medical condition
- Schizoaffective disorder
- Bipolar affective disorder manic episode with psychotic symptoms
- Depressive episode with psychotic symptoms
- Delusional disorder
- Acute and transient psychotic disorder
- Paranoid personality disorder.

Medical conditions to be excluded when evaluating a patient with first episode psychosis include:

- Temporal lobe epilepsy
- Toxic drug reaction
- Systemic lupus erythematosus
- Infections – limbic encephalitis, subacute sclerosing encephalitis, neurosyphilis and HIV disease
- CNS neoplasm, cerebral trauma
- Cerebrovascular disease (late-onset schizophrenia)
- Huntington's disease
- Metabolic disorders – electrolyte imbalance, hypoglycaemia, hepatic or renal disease
- Endocrine disorders – hyper- and hypothyroidism, Addison's disease, hyper- and hypoparathyroidism
- Demyelinating disease, such as multiple sclerosis and metachromatic dystrophy.

Persistent delusional disorder

- Rule out physical causes, e.g., head injury, epilepsy, CNS infection
- Substance-induced delusional disorder, e.g., alcohol, hallucinogens, stimulants
- Schizophrenia
- Mood disorder with delusions
- Elderly patients (late paraphrenia)
- Paranoid personality disorder
- Obsessive–compulsive disorder (OCD)
- Body dysmorphic disorder
- Hypochondriasis.

Mania

- Schizophrenia
- Schizoaffective disorder

- Drug or alcohol induced mania
- Medical disorder induced mania
- Delirium or acute confusional state
- Agitated depression in the elderly
- Obsessive–compulsive disorder or other anxiety disorders
- Circadian rhythm disorders
- Puerperal psychosis (in women)
- Dementia, especially frontal (in the elderly).

Organic causes of manic and hypomanic symptoms:

- Metabolic disturbance – postoperative states, postinfection states, hyperthyroidism, Cushing's disease, Addison's disease
- Infection – influenza, neurosyphilis, AIDS (HIV), herpes simplex encephalitis
- Neurological conditions – epilepsy, post-cerebrovascular accident, multiple sclerosis, right temporal seizure focus
- Neoplasm – parasagittal meningioma, suprasellar craniopharyngioma, tumour of the floor of the fourth ventricle
- Illicit drugs associated with manic symptoms – amphetamines, cocaine, hallucinogens and opiates
- Medications associated with manic symptoms – antidepressants, isoniazid, levodopa, methyl phenidate hydrochloride, procyclidine hydrochloride, bromocriptine mesilate, corticosteroids, cimetidine, ciclosporin

Depression

- Mood disorder due to a general medical condition
- Substance-induced mood disorder – alcohol, amphetamine, heroin, cocaine, etc.
- Bipolar affective disorder
- Dysthymia
- Consider stress-related disorders, such as adjustment disorder, grief reaction, PTSD
- Dementia
- Anxiety disorders, such as social phobias, OCD, panic disorder
- Schizophrenia (negative symptoms)
- Personality disorders, such as borderline PD.

Medical conditions inducing mood disorder:

- Metabolic – iron-deficiency anaemia, niacin deficiency (pellagra), hypercalcaemia
- Infective – encephalitis, post-viral, hepatitis, infectious mononucleosis, HIV

- Neurological – post-stroke, Parkinson's disease, multiple sclerosis, intracranial tumours (e.g., frontal)
- Non-metastasis manifestation of neoplasm, e.g., pancreatic carcinoma
- Endocrine disorders: hypothyroidism, Cushing's syndrome, Addison's disease hyperparathyroidism
- Iatrogenic – reserpine, propranolol hydrochloride, alpha methyldopa, corticosteroids; effects of chemotherapeutic agents, such as vincristine sulfate and interferons; whole-brain radiotherapy.

Anxiety disorders

- Medical disorders causing anxiety symptoms – thyrotoxicosis, hypoglycaemia, phaeochromocytoma, temporal lobe epilepsy, anaemia, asthma, cardiac arrhythmias and carcinoid tumours, hypoxia, sepsis
- Medication inducing anxiety symptoms – bronchodilators, antihypertensives, antiarrhythmics, anticonvulsants, thyroxine sodium, antiparkinsonian agents, antidepressants, antipsychotics, Antabuse (disulfiram) reactions
- Affective disorder – depression, depression with agitated features
- Consider all other anxiety disorders – agoraphobia, social phobia, specific phobia, panic disorder, generalized anxiety disorder, mixed anxiety and depressive disorder, OCD, acute stress reaction, PTSD, adjustment reaction
- Substance misuse – alcohol withdrawal symptoms, drug withdrawal symptoms
- Prodromal symptom of schizophrenia
- Early stage of dementia.

Social phobias

- Agoraphobias
- Panic disorder
- Depressive disorder
- Generalized anxiety disorder
- Avoidant personality disorder
- Social inadequacy
- Schizophrenia.

Obsessive–compulsive disorder

- Normal thoughts, worries (but recurrent)
- Anankastic personality disorder
- Depressive disorder
- Hypochondriasis

- Phobias
- Schizophrenia
- Body dysmorphic disorder.

Post-traumatic stress disorder

- Adjustment disorder
- Acute stress reaction
- Enduring personality change after a catastrophic event
- Depressive/mood disorder
- Generalized anxiety disorders
- Phobias
- Panic disorder
- Substance-induced disorders
- Obsessive–compulsive disorder
- Schizophrenia or other associated psychosis.

Anorexia nervosa

- Weight loss due to a general medical condition: especially gastrointestinal (GI) disorders, such as inflammatory bowel disease, malabsorption syndrome and occult malignancy
- Vomiting secondary to gastric outlet obstruction
- Brain tumour
- HIV
- Loss of appetite may be secondary to drugs, e.g., selective serotonin (5-hydroxytryptamine) reuptake inhibitors (SSRIs), amphetamines
- Bulimia nervosa (50% of anorexia suffers also meet the criteria for bulimia nervosa)
- Depressive disorder
- Obsessive–compulsive disorder
- Schizophrenia.

Bulimia nervosa

- Upper GI disorders
- Depressive disorder
- Obsessive-compulsive disorder
- Personality disorders
- Drug-related increased appetite (antipsychotics, antidepressants especially tricyclic antidepressants, mood stabilizers)
- Causes of recurrent overeating, such as Kleine–Levin syndrome.

Dementia

- Depressive disorder (pseudo-dementia)
- Delirium
- Drugs
- Amnesic syndromes
- Learning disability
- Late-onset psychotic disorder
- Normal ageing.

Alzheimer's dementia

- Non-Alzheimer's dementia
- Vascular dementia/multi-infarct dementia
- Lewy body dementia
- Fronto-temporal dementia
- Subcortical dementias, such as Parkinson's disease, Huntington's disease
- Metabolic toxic dementias, such as hypothyroidism, hyperparathyroidism, vitamin B12 and folate deficiency
- Infections, e.g., syphilis, HIV, chronic meningitis.

Schizotypal disorder

- Autism
- Asperger's syndrome
- Chronic substance misuse
- Personality disorders, such as schizoid, paranoid and borderline types
- Expressive language disorder.

Asperger's syndrome

- Schizophrenia – paranoid, simple
- Personality disorders – schizoid, avoidant, anankastic and dissocial
- Attention deficit hyperactivity disorders
- Anxiety states – selective mutism, social phobias, panic disorder, generalized anxiety disorders
- Obsessive–compulsive disorder.

Borderline personality disorder

- Organic personality disorder – secondary to a general medical condition, e.g., cerebral neoplasms especially in frontal and parietal lobes
- Mood disorders – depressive disorder with atypical features
- Psychotic disorders
- Other personality disorders, such as antisocial PD, histrionic PD, dependent PD types.

5

Aetiological formulation

By the end of each clinical assessment, every trainee is expected to be able to address the question.

'Why has this patient developed this disorder at this point in their life?'

Remember the 3 Ps:

- Predisposing factors
- Precipitating factors
- Perpetuating factors.

Consider biological, psychological and social causes and cross-tabulate these with predisposing, precipitating and perpetuating factors (see Table 5.1)

Candidates are not expected to 'fill in' every one of the boxes in Table 5.1, but you will have had to think about each.

For an example using schizophrenia see Table 5.2.

TABLE 5.1 Structure of an aetiological formulation

Aetiological factors	Biological factors	Psychological factors	Social factors
Predisposing			
Precipitating			
Perpetuating			

TABLE 5.2 Example of a dimensional approach to the aetiology of schizophrenia

Aetiological factors	Biological factors	Psychological factors	Social factors
Predisposing	Genetic risk	Schizotypal personality	Urban birth
Precipitating	Cannabis misuse	High expressed emotion	Life events
Perpetuating	Non-compliance with treatment	Poor insight	Homelessness

Commonly identified aetiological factors

- Recent stressful life events
- Non-compliance with medications
- Non-engagement with services
- Lack of insight
- Substance misuse
- Co-morbid physical illnesses
- Social isolation
- Poor financial support, lack of employment, housing
- Poor premorbid adjustments
- Previous history of mental illness
- Family history of mental illness
- Recent bereavement (elderly)
- Sensory deprivation (elderly).

The other aetiological risk factors specifically to be looked for in the common psychiatric conditions given are outlined below.

Schizophrenia

- Genetic risk – positive family history.

Environmental insults in early development

- Perinatal trauma – obstetric complications
- Perinatal infection – prenatal exposure to influenza
- Urban settings – city birth
- Degree of urbanization at birth.

Childhood period

- Delayed motor developmental milestones, including delayed walking
- Preference for solitary play
- Lower educational test scores at different levels, such as age 8, 11 and 15 years
- Low premorbid IQ.

Others

- Children of migrants
- Substance abuse – heavy cannabis intake
- Recent stressful life events

- High expressed emotion (emotional over-involvement, critical comments and hostility)
- City/rural areas.

Depression

In childhood

- Genetic risk
- Parental loss
- Emotional, physical or sexual abuse
- Perceived lack of parental warmth, acceptance and affection
- Disturbed family environment.

In adolescence

- Early onset anxiety disorder
- Early onset conduct disorder
- Presence of neurotic personality traits
- Low self-esteem
- Low educational attainment.

In adulthood

- Stressful life events and ongoing psychosocial stressors
- Poor social support
- Personal history of mood disorder
- Marital problems
- Physical illness
- Substance abuse, e.g., alcohol
- Non-compliance with medication
- Unemployment
- Loss of role
- Negative cognitive style – learned helplessness and Beck's negative cognitive triad
- Lack of perceived control over future
- Positive family history
- Personality – obsessional, dependent, anxious and borderline traits in the personality.

Brown and Harris vulnerability factors

- Having three children under 14 years of age at home

- Lack of paid employment
- Lack of a confidant relationship.

Mania

- Family history
- Non-compliance with medication
- Intercurrent substance misuse
- Recent life event
- Social rhythm disruption – new shift work, recent delivery of a baby, sleep deprivation secondary to long haul flights.

Anorexia nervosa

Predisposing factors

- Personal events – emotional, physical and sexual childhood abuse
- Vulnerable personality – obsessional and impulsive borderline traits in the personality
- Family conflict – enmeshment, over-involvement, scapegoat
- Any psychiatric disorder (depression, anxiety, deliberate self-harm) in the patient
- Positive family history of affective disorder
- Stressful life events
- Social factors – Western society and cult of thinness
- Genetic constitutional – whether vulnerable to weight loss or disordered 5-hydroxytryptamine (serotonin) system
- Early life experiences – parental loss and separation
- Personality traits.

Precipitating factors

- Recent stressful life events
- Treatment issues – recent alteration in drugs or therapies.

Perpetuating factors

- Personality issues
- Family factors
- Primary or secondary gain.

Alcoholism

- Male sex
- Occupation – journalists, doctors, vets, publicans
- Early drinking, life-long
- Positive family history of alcoholism or depression
- Childhood abuse or neglect
- Co-morbid drug misuse
- Previous periods of inpatient or outpatient detoxification
- Relationship and work difficulties
- Forensic history
- Antisocial personality traits/disorder
- Conduct disorder during childhood
- Impulsivity, angry and aggressive personality traits
- Psychiatric history of anxiety, social phobia and depression.

Post-traumatic stress disorder

- Female sex
- Afro-Caribbean/Hispanic
- Lower socioeconomic class
- Lower education
- Presence of neurotic traits
- Presence of low self-esteem
- History of previous traumatic events or childhood experiences
- Past history of mood disorders/anxiety disorders
- Family history of mood disorders/anxiety disorder.

Alzheimer's dementia

- Older age
- Female gender
- Positive family history
- Past history of head injury
- Low educational status
- Down's syndrome.

Vascular dementia

- Older age
- Female gender

- History of diabetes mellitus
- History of hypertension and other vascular disease
- Atrial fibrillation
- History of depression
- Cigarette smoking.

6

Investigations

Types of investigation

- Physical/medical
- Psychological
- Social.

Physical investigations

- Think, in advance, which investigations are appropriate for your case.
- Use your common sense.
- Mention the investigations that you carry out in your routine day-to-day practice, and those that are appropriate and relevant to your case.

Blood

- Full blood count (FBC)
- B12 and folate levels
- Liver function tests (LFTs)
- Urea and electrolytes (U&Es)
- Creatinine
- Thyroid function tests (TFT)
- Blood sugar.

Where there is suspicion of drug or alcohol dependency, check mean corpuscular volume (MCV), and toxicology screening may be added.

Special tests for selected cases should only be carried out if the history and physical examination warrants it. These tests include:

- VDRL (Venereal Disease Research Laboratory)
- Hepatitis B, hepatitis C
- HIV (human immunodeficiency virus).

Urine

- Urine drug screen
- Mid-stream urine – microscopy, culture and sensitivity in elderly patients and where history suggests.

Imaging

- Chest X-ray (CXR) – elderly patients, and only where examination and history suggests morbid respiratory and cardiovascular conditions
- Electrocardiogram (ECG) – only for specific cases (elderly patients and for patients on high-dose antipsychotics, special populations with cardiac problems)
- Electroencephalogram (EEG) – requires justification on the grounds of diagnostic need
- Computed tomography (CT) – requires justification on the grounds of diagnostic need
- Magnetic resonance imaging (MRI) – only for specific cases
- Other investigations as dictated by findings on physical examination.

Psychological investigations

- Psychometric testing/neuropsychological assessment if you suspect dementia, cognitive impairment, organic psychiatric illness or learning disability
- Rating scales to establish baselines (mood rating scales, anxiety and depression rating scales)
- Personality assessment (only for specific cases)

The following types of self-monitoring can be requested if appropriate:

- Mood diary
- Eating or drinking diary
- Activities diary.

Social investigations

Different sources of information include:

- Collateral history from:
  - Partners
  - Relatives

– Friends
– Carers (formal and informal) with the patient's consent
● Liaising with:
  – GP and primary care staff, e.g., the district nurse
  – Nursing team involved in the patient's care and in the unit
  – Other members of the multidisciplinary team, such as the community psychiatric nurse, social worker, occupational therapist and other professionals
● Notes:
  – Previous medical notes/psychiatric notes
  – Nursing notes
  – Previous discharge summaries
  – Care programme approach (CPA) forms and old written care plans
● Reports
  – Occupational therapist's assessment report
  – Social worker's assessment report
  – Community psychiatric nurse's/care-coordinator's report
  – Other relevant report
  – School reports (child and learning disability cases)
  – Court report
  – Police reports
  – Forensic reports.

7

Management plan

As part of your WPBA preparation, you should write out typical structured management plans for common conditions, such as schizophrenia, affective disorders, neurotic disorders, substance misuse and eating disorders. The management plan should be tailored according to the individual case.

The management plan should be divided into:

- Immediate/short term management
- Long-term management.

Remember:

- 'Biopsychosocial model' (physical, psychological and social)
  - Psychopharmacological treatment
  - Psychotherapeutic interventions
  - Psychosocial interventions
- Multidisciplinary team approach.

Immediate/short-term management

Medical

Psychopharmacological/physical

- Medication (antipsychotics, antidepressants, mood stabilizers, benzo-diazepines and medications for physical health problems) – discussed in detail in the latter part of this book
- Electroconvulsive therapy (ECT) – if appropriate.

Nursing

Nursing assessment involving:
- Observation of behaviour

- Monitoring of biological functions, such as sleep pattern and appetite
- Checking compliance with medication and personal hygiene
- Providing emotional and practical support (if necessary in the unit)
- Encouraging the patient to attend ward activities
- Different levels of observation according to the patient's current mental state
- Referral to day hospital
- Routine urine and drug screening for selected cases
- Comprehensive risk assessment.

Psychological

Please mention the following only if appropriate to your case:

- Advice and structured counselling
- Psychoeducation for the patient and the family
- Compliance therapy
- Insight-oriented therapy
- Supportive psychotherapy
- Behaviour therapy (child psychiatry, learning disability and selected cases)
- Drug education/motivational programme (drug and alcohol misuse)
- Involve the psychologist to identify and develop successful coping strategies for both the patient and the relatives and to identify the mode of psychological support that patients may require on a long-term basis, including:
  - Cognitive behavioural therapy (CBT) – individual and group
  - Family therapy assessment
  - Psychodynamic – individual, group therapy assessment
  - Cognitive analytical therapy (CAT)
  - Dialectical behavioural therapy (DBT).

Social

- Involve occupational therapists to carry out occupational therapy assessments including home assessments:
  - To determine activities of daily living (ADL) skills, level of functioning and to ascertain the level of support needed
  - To enhance their life skills training, social skills training, problem-solving skills and relaxation techniques
  - To focus on rehabilitation, mainly vocational rehabilitation, to regain their lost skills and to build up their confidence.
- Involve a social worker and social services who could help with:
  - Community care assessment (needs assessment), assessment of financial

status and carer's assessment, if necessary, and organise an appropriate 'care package' that addresses the needs of both patient and carers.
- Support regarding placement, benefits, employment and leisure activities
- In elderly and learning disability patients – will determine the need for homecare provision such as a home carer, 'meals-on-wheels', sitting services, day centre attendance and respite care, and for long-term placement.
- Involve community psychiatric nurses (CPNs):
  - To monitor the mental state in the community, compliance with medications, efficacy and tolerability of medications
  - To provide additional support such as anxiety management, stress management, relaxation training and relapse prevention work
  - To identify early-relapse indicators.
- Predischarge care programme approach (CPA) meetings and care plan – discharge the patient with adequate community support and a care plan.

Long-term management

The long-term management would focus on:

- Relapse prevention
- Rehabilitation
- Quality-of-life improvement.

Biological

Mnemonic – 4 Cs:

- Continue medications – maintenance therapy and outpatient follow-up
- Community psychiatric nurse or care coordinator monitoring in the community
- Crisis and contingency plans – assertive outreach team, 24-hour crisis access team (depends on available local resources)
- Care programme approach – regular reviews, care plan still in place.

Psychological

- Individual and group CBT
- Family therapy
- Individual/group psychotherapy
- Attendance at day hospital.

Relapse prevention strategies include identifying early warning signs to prevent, identify and intervene for possible precipitant and identifying care pathways.

Social

Mnemonic – 8 Ss:

- Self-help manuals
- Self-help groups
- Support groups
- Support through day centres/drop-ins
- Supported education
- Supported employment
- Supported housing and other kinds of placements include independent flats, warden-controlled shelter accommodation, sheltered-plus accommodation, residential placement, residential elderly mentally infirm (EMI) placement, nursing home placement
- Service interventions – to be increased, such as increased contact with key workers and improved liaison with primary care services
- Voluntary agencies
- Patient advocacy services.

Schizophrenia

First episode schizophrenia

First episode patients:

- The treatment should focus on bringing acute symptoms under control and establishing a long-range treatment plan.
- For first episode patients, dosage recommendations tend to be considerably lower but some patients may require higher doses than recommended.
- Some degree of response is expected within the first 1–2 weeks, though the ultimate degree of response can take considerably longer. As a general rule, some clinically significant improvement should be observed within the *first 2 weeks*, and up to 50% of the ultimate improvement may be seen within *4 weeks*.
- If a reasonable degree of improvement is observed, the following steps should be taken:
  1. Management of adverse effects, if any
  2. Initiation and planning of appropriate psychosocial and rehabilitative services
  3. Family psychoeducation
  4. Implementation of successful follow-up care.
- The maintenance treatment is recommended for 1–2 years following a first episode.
- For patients presenting with a first episode psychosis, substance abuse is an important differential diagnosis to be considered, and urine-screening tests should be conducted routinely.
- First episode schizophrenia outcome – 87% achieve remission at median period of 11 weeks.

Relapse rates

- Relapse (Lieberman et al, 1996; Robinson et al, 1999):
  - 16% by year 1
  - 54% by year 2
  - 82% by year 5.
- After each relapse, 1 in 6 did not remit.
- Suicide occurs in 11% of schizophrenic patients.
- Patients in good remission for long periods still have an average relapse rate of 75% within 1–2 years of discontinuation of medication.
- Research evidence also suggests that approximately 16–20% of patients will relapse during the course of a year with adequate pharmacological treatment.
- When non-compliance is an additional factor, then as many as 40–50% of patients may experience a relapse within a year.

- The abrupt discontinuation of antipsychotics leads to a cumulative relapse rate of 46% at 6 months and 56% at 2 years.

Maintenance treatment

- Following recovery from a first episode of psychosis associated with a schizophrenic illness, 1–2 years is usually the recommendation and the patient should be maintained on a standard dose of antipsychotic medication.
- For multi-episode patients, these recommendations do not generally exceed 5 years.
- If further deterioration of functional capacity occurs with each episode, the recommendations are towards longer intervals of maintenance treatment.
- Meta-analytic studies of six double-blind randomized controlled trials of low-dose antipsychotic maintenance indicated that low-dose therapy is not as effective as a standard dose in preventing relapse (Barbui et al, 1999).
- Randomized controlled trials on high-dose antipsychotics did not show any significant advantage over a standard dose.
- For patients with history of non-compliance, the use of depot drugs should be considered as this can enhance compliance.

Inadequate response to antipsychotics

The following steps should be taken:

- Consider adherence issues and check the compliance by measuring the blood levels (if possible), which helps to not only confirm the degree of compliance but also to identify individuals with unusually low blood levels despite adequate dosage.
- Review the psychiatric diagnosis.
- Review the past treatment.
- Rule out substance abuse.
- Rule out co-morbidity, such as affective disorder.
- Identify psychosocial stressors, to reduce them and help the patient to cope with them.

Next steps:

- Wait in the hope that the patient is slow to respond (questionable).
- Increase the dose.
- Switch to a different antipsychotic agent.
- Add adjunctive pharmacological treatment.

If the adherence is doubtful or known to be poor, then investigate the reasons for it:

- If the patient is *confused or disorganized*, then:
  - Simplify the drug regimen
  - Consider compliance aids
  - Reduce the anticholinergic dosage as it can worsen the confusion.
- If the patient lacks *adequate insight*, then consider:
  - Compliance therapy
  - Depot antipsychotic.
- If the patient does not seem to *tolerate* then:
  - Discuss with the patient
  - Consider switch to acceptable drug with lesser side effects.

Treatment-resistant schizophrenia

Less restrictive definition of treatment-resistant schizophrenia (TRS):

> Lack of a satisfactory clinical improvement despite the sequential use of the recommended doses for 6 to 8 weeks of at least two antipsychotic drugs at least one of which should be an atypical.

> (NICE, 2002)

Pharmacological strategies

Antipsychotic drugs

- Ensure adequate trial of atypical antipsychotics (recommended dosage for adequate duration, e.g., 6–8 weeks).
- Switch to another class of antipsychotic – either second generation atypical or first generation typical antipsychotics. If a patient has been on a conventional agent, and there is reason to switch then a new generation antipsychotic should be considered. The choice of drug and dosage will also be influenced by an evaluation of past treatment response. If a patient has a history of responding well to a particular agent then that medication should be considered a first choice unless other factors come into play.
- If all these measures fail, then consider clozapine.

Clozapine

- Clozapine is not recommended unless patients have failed on two other antipsychotic drugs.
- The average dose recommended is approximately 450 mg/day but the response is usually seen in the range 150–900 mg/day.
- Plasma levels above a threshold of 350–400 ng/ml are associated with the highest likelihood of response and a trial duration of 3–6 months should achieve some clinically significant improvement in psychopathology.

- An adequate trial of 6–12 months should be done with clozapine, and the evidence suggests an advantage to longer treatment with clozapine.
- Research evidence suggests that clozapine seemed to:
  - Have specific positive effects on hostility, aggression, disorganization and affective symptoms in schizoaffective disorder
  - Improve cognitive functions, such as attention and verbal fluency
  - Reduce the rate of suicidality
  - Reduce the rate of smoking
  - Reduce rates of relapse and rehospitalization.

Clozapine augmentation – suggested options:

- Amisulpride augmentation (400–800 mg/day)
- Add sulpiride (400 mg/day)
- Add risperidone (2 mg/day)
- Add lamotrigine (25–300 mg/day)
- Add omega 3-triglycerides (2–3 g EPA daily)
- Lithium augmentation.

Other adjunctive treatments

- Mood stabilizers or anticonvulsants such as sodium valproate and carbamazepine are used more frequently than lithium for patients with impulsivity, excitement and aggressive behaviour, and they are more likely to improve with these drugs.
- Carbamazepine is a potent inducer of hepatic enzymes and concomitant administration can cause a 50% or greater reduction in blood levels of antipsychotics medications.
- Antidepressants, such as selective serotonin (5-hydroxytryptamine) re-uptake inhibitors (SSRIs) and tricyclic antidepressants have been widely used as adjunctive treatments but primarily to treat co-morbid depression or post-psychotic depression.
- ECT is another adjunctive treatment, and it can be effective as an adjunct to clozapine in treatment refractory patients.
- The benzodiazepines are used to treat agitation, anxiety and irritability. The therapeutic effects develop rapidly but the positive effects are modest, transient and also diminish after a few weeks.

Negative symptoms

The treatment of negative symptoms is a major challenge that most clinicians are facing.

Conditions that may *mimic negative symptoms* are:

- Depression – 'True flat effect' is seen in individuals with negative symptoms but not in the case of depression
- Antipsychotic drug-induced parkinsonian side effects
- Effects of chronic institutionalization
- Withdrawal in response to a frightening psychotic experience.

The pharmacological strategies for the treatment of negative symptoms include:

- Dopaminergic agents – levodopa, amphetamine, bromocriptine mesilate
- Serotonergic agents – fluoxetine hydrochloride, fluvoxamine malate
- Noradrenergic agents – propranalol hydrochloride, clonidine hydrochloride
- Glutaminergic agents – cycloserine, glycine.

Cognitive symptoms

The new generation antipsychotic medications can improve cognitive functioning to a measurable and statistically significant degree.

- Clozapine has been associated with improvements in executive function, verbal fluency, and fine motor function.
- Risperidone has been associated with improvement in attention and executive functions.

Common side effects of antipsychotic medications

Typical antipsychotics

- Sedation, dizziness, postural hypotension
- Anticholinergic side effects, such as dry mouth, constipation, blurred vision, urinary retention and confusion in the elderly
- Endocrine effects, including increased appetite, weight gain, diminished libido, impaired ejaculation, amenorrhoea, galactorrhoea
- Extrapyramidal side effects, such as akathisia, acute dystonia, parkinsonism, tardive dyskinesia.

Atypical antipsychotics

- *Olanzapine* – sedation, weight gain, dizziness, postural hypotension, peripheral oedema, anticholinergic side effects such as dry mouth, constipation, hypotension, impaired glucose tolerance and asymptomatic increase in liver enzymes
- *Risperidone* – insomnia, agitation, anxiety, headache, extrapyramidal side effects, postural hypotension especially at the beginning of the treatment, drowsiness, dizziness, nausea, abdominal pain, weight gain, sexual disturbances

- *Quetiapine fumarate* – dizziness, drowsiness, dyspepsia, postural hypotension, weight gain, constipation, dry mouth, hypertension, tachycardia
- *Amisulpride* – insomnia, anxiety, agitation, anticholinergic side effects such as constipation, dry mouth, increased prolactin levels causing amenorrhoea, galactorrhoea, loss of libido, breast engorgement
- *Clozapine* – sedation, constipation, dizziness, postural hypotension, transient tachycardia, hyperthermia (fever), hypertension, weight gain, hypersalivation, neutropenia/agranulocytosis, seizures
- *Aripiprazole* – constipation, akathisia, headache, nausea, vomiting, stomach upset, agitation, anxiety, insomnia, sleepiness, lightheadedness, tremor
- *Zotepine* – dry mouth, constipation, dyspepsia, tachycardia, headache, agitation, anxiety, QT interval prolongation, weight gain, sexual dysfunction.

Dosage ranges are given for a number of drugs in Tables 7.1 and 7.2.

Advantages of newer atypicals over typical antipsychotics

- Lower propensity to cause extrapyramidal side effects
- Lower risk of tardive dyskinesia
- Superior efficacy against negative symptoms, depressive symptoms and cognitive symptoms.

As a result of these factors, there could be:

- Enhancement of quality of life
- Improved rates of compliance
- Improved functioning as well as a greater likelihood of participating in psychosocial and vocational therapies.

Management of adverse effects

- Sedation:
  - Giving medication all or largely at night can be helpful
  - Dose reduction or changing to a less sedating medication are alternative strategies
- Orthostatic hypotension:
  - Gradual dosage escalation can be helpful
  - The patient should be instructed to rise slowly from a seated or prone position
  - Switching to another medication is also helpful
- Extrapyramidal side effects:
  - Reduction in dosage
  - Switching to another antipsychotic agent, e.g., olanzapine, quetiapine fumarate, clozapine

TABLE **7.1** Dosage ranges for antipsychotic and other drugs

Drug names	Usual daily dose range (mg)
Typical antipsychotics	
Chlorpromazine	50–1000
Haloperidol	1–20
Trifluoperazine	5–30
Flupenthixol	6–18
Zuclopenthixol	20–150
Sulpiride	200–2400
Atypical antipsychotics	
Olanzapine	5–20
Risperidone	2–8
Quetiapine fumarate	300–750
Clozapine	200–450
Amisulpride	50–300 (negative symptoms)
	400–1200 (positive symptoms)
Zotepine	150–450
Ziprasidone	80–160
Dopamine stabilizer	
Aripiprazole	5–30
Depot medications	
Zuclopenthixol acetate	50–150; IM every 2–3 days
Fluphenazine decanoate	12.5–100; IM every 2 weeks
Flupenthixol decanoate	20–400; IM every 2–4 weeks
Haloperidol decanoate	50–300; IM every 4 weeks
Zuclopenthixol decanoate	200–400; IM every 2–4 weeks
Pipotiazine decanoate	50–200; IM every 4 weeks
Risperidone long-acting injection	25–50; every 2 weeks

TABLE **7.2** Dosage recommendations for newer antipsychotics

Drug	First episode (mg)	Multiple episode (mg)
Olanzapine	5–10	10–20
Risperidone	2–4	4–10
Quetiapine fumarate	200–400	400–750
Amisulpride	30–400	400–1200
Clozapine	100–200	400–900

- Use of anticholinergic agents, such as procyclidine hydrochloride, orphenadrine, biperiden, trihexyphenidyl hydrochloride
- Acute dystonic reaction – intramuscular medication, either anticholinergic or antihistaminic
- Akathisia:
  - Reduce the dose or slow down the increase of potential causative agent
  - Consider use of lower potency agents
  - Beta-blocker such as propranolol hydrochloride may be helpful

- Benzodiazepines such as clonazepam, diazepam and lorazepam can also be helpful
- Tardive dyskinesia:
  - The incidence of tardive dyskinesia was approximately 5% per year of drug exposure with relatively consistent risk occurring for the first 8–10 years of treatment
  - The risk has been shown to be five times higher in elderly patients treated with conventional antipsychotic drugs
  - Drug discontinuation or switching to a different medication (atypical antipsychotics) can be helpful
- Weight gain:
  - Encourage moderate physical exercise
  - Encourage healthy diet, avoiding high calorie foods
  - Involve dietician if necessary
  - Use lowest therapeutic dose
  - Introduce medication increases slowly
  - Switch to medications that have less effect on weight gain
  - Use adjunctive pharmacological treatments, such as orlistat, methyl phenidate hydrochloride or sibutramine
- Endocrine effects – hyperprolactinaemia:
  - It is reversible upon stopping medication
  - It can be associated with painful breasts, swollen breasts, amenorrhoea and galactorrhoea, predispose women to cardiovascular disease and osteoporosis and, in men, there is reduced steroidogenesis and spermatogenesis and sexual dysfunction
  - Consider reduction in dose if the patient's mental state is stable
  - Newer generation medications tend to have much less effect on prolactin, with risperidone being the most likely and quetiapine fumarate and clozapine the least likely to cause prolactin elevation
  - Asymptomatic hyperprolactinaemia in itself does not warrant change to medication
- Sexual dysfunction:
  - Erectile dysfunction, ejaculatory disturbances and loss of libido can occur in men and diminished libido and anorgasmia can occur in women with use of antipsychotics
  - Reducing dosages or switching medications is sometimes necessary
  - Consider switching to alternative agents, such as low-dose olanzapine, quetiapine fumarate and clozapine
  - Imipramine has been used for treating retrograde ejaculation
  - Yohimbine hydrochloride, cyproheptadine hydrochloride and sildenafil citrate have been helpful for some patients with erectile dysfunction
- Metabolic syndrome:
  - Core features:

a. Obesity – central or upper body
b. Insulin resistance or hyperinsulinaemia
c. Dyslipidaemia
d. Impaired glucose tolerance or type 2 diabetes mellitus
e. Hypertension
- Metabolic syndrome is identified more in patients on atypical antipsychotics, but it can occur in patients on typical antipsychotics as well
- Lifestyle and risk factor modification, such as reduced dietary fat content, increased physical activity, avoiding smoking, reduced alcohol intake, monitoring weight, monitoring metabolic markers (e.g., glucose and lipid profile), can reduce the morbidity and mortality rate, improve the level of function and provide a better quality of life.

Issues of non-compliance

Factors contributing to non-compliance in schizophrenia

- Patient-related:
  - Lack of insight
  - Lack of education about the illness
  - Symptom severity
  - Denial
  - Delusional beliefs
  - Co-morbid conditions
- Treatment related:
  - Medication side effects, particularly extrapyramidal side effects (EPSEs), weight gain and sexual dysfunction
  - Complex prescribing regimens
- Environmental factors:
  - Inadequate social support
  - Stigma.

Compliance aids (e.g., Medidose system)

The ultimate aim should be to promote independent living, perhaps with the patient filling in their own compliance aid, having first been given support and training, but the patient should be clearly motivated to adhere to the prescribed treatment.

Psychosocial management strategies

Psychosocial treatment should be provided to patients, families and to significant others involved in their care. The approach should be tailored to the special needs of individual patients.

Psycho-education

Individual psycho-education to be offered to the patient regarding:

- The nature of the illness
- The characteristic symptoms of the illness
- Available treatment options
- The therapeutic effects and side effects of medications
- Discussion of the longer treatment plan
- Identifying early warning signs of relapse.

Compliance therapy

This consists of 4–6 sessions based on motivational interviewing and cognitive psycho-educational approaches to psychotic symptoms. It also emphasizes the importance of the treatment alliance and patient participation.

Cognitive behavioural therapy

Individual and group therapies employing well-specified combinations of support, education, cognitive and behavioural approaches, social-skills training approaches. It also enhances other targeted problems such as medication non-compliance. Cognitive behavioural therapy in addition to drug treatment reduces persistent positive symptoms.

The *cognitive* components involve:

- Identifying links between thoughts, emotions and behaviour and identifying automatic thoughts
- Hypothesis testing about abnormal beliefs and reframing attributions
- Identifying and enhancing coping strategies.

The *behavioural* elements involve:

- Symptom monitoring
- Use of diary
- Distraction techniques, which focus strategies for hallucinatory experiences
- Graded task assignment
- Anxiety management and relaxation techniques.

Family therapy

Family psychosocial interventions usually last for at least 9 months and provide a combination of:

- Education about the illness and its management
- Family support

- Focusing on strategies to reduce stress within the family
- Maintaining reasonable expectations for the patient's performance
- Crisis intervention.

The various approaches commonly focus on positive areas of family functioning and increasing family structure and stability through problem solving, goal setting and cognitive restructuring.

- It should also be offered to non-family caregivers.
- It should not be restricted to patients whose families are identified as having high levels of expressed emotion.
- The family interventions are known to be effective in reducing relapse.

Other approaches

- Motivational intervention techniques can reduce street drug use and enhance treatment compliance.
- Cognitive remediation in chronic schizophrenia aims to treat patients on specific neuropsychological tasks, and it reduces cognitive deficits in chronic schizophrenia.
- Social skills training uses learning theory principles to break complex repertoires down into simpler tasks, subjects them to corrective learning and applies them in real-life settings, thereby helping the patient to regain and improve social skills.
- Vocational rehabilitation includes prevocational training, transitional employment, supported employment, vocational counselling and education services (job clubs, rehabilitation counselling, post-employment services).

Other service provision

- Day hospitals
  - These can provide an alternative to inpatient care in certain situations.
  - They are semi-residential structures in which short- and medium-term therapeutic and rehabilitative programmes are carried out.
  - They are intended for patients with subacute psychiatric disorders who are in need of drug therapy, psychotherapy and/or rehabilitative therapy.
  - Their purpose is to avoid, as far as possible, the need for a full-time hospital stay during periods of patient relapse or inability to cope, and to limit the duration of such a stay if it becomes a necessity.
- Assertive community treatment programmes should be targeted to individuals at high risk for repeated hospitalizations or who have been difficult to retain in active treatment with more traditional types of services.

- The care programme approach (CPA) plays a major role in:
  - Assessing the patient's clinical and other needs
  - Formulating a 'written care plan' with a planned programme of care
  - Identifying a care manager or care coordinator to maintain contact with the patient
  - Arranging discharge planning CPA meeting
  - Coordinating all the members involved in the patient's care
  - Arranging regular reviews once every 6 months with all members involved in the patient's care.
- Community mental health teams (CMHT) also provide effective treatment with comprehensive assessment of individual patients, provide support and monitor the patient for early warning signs of relapse.

Monitoring

Recommended monitoring for newer antipsychotics

- Baseline:
  - Full blood count
  - Urea and electrolytes
  - Blood lipids
  - Liver function tests
  - Glycosylated haemoglobin
  - Weight
  - Blood pressure
  - Electrocardiogram (ECG; optional)
- Glycosylated haemoglobin, urea and electrolytes, liver function tests should be repeated after 6 months and then yearly
- Creatinine phosphokinase if neuroleptic malignant syndrome is suspected
- Electrocardiogram when maintenance dose is reached
- Electroencephalogram (EEG), if myoclonus or seizures occur
- Prolactin level, if symptoms of hyperprolactinaemia occur
- Blood lipids – after 3 months and then yearly.

Recommended monitoring for clozapine

- Perform baseline blood tests (white cell count and differential count) before starting clozapine
- Full blood count – weekly for the first 18 weeks, then at least every 2 weeks for 1 year and monthly thereafter
- Daily monitoring of pulse, temperature and blood pressure for at least the first 2 weeks after initiating the treatment.

Additional monitoring requirements:

- Baseline – weight, glycosylated haemoglobin, liver function tests
- One month – weight, plasma glucose
- Three months – weight, glycosylated haemoglobin
- Six months – weight, glycosylated haemoglobin, liver function tests
- Twelve months – weight, glycosylated haemoglobin.

Consider also use of ECG where available and also monitor plasma lipids.

Monitoring physical health
All patients with schizophrenia who are on long-term treatment with antipsychotics should have an annual review, normally in primary care, to ensure that the following are assessed each year:

- Weight
- Smoking status and alcohol use
- Blood pressure
- Plasma glucose levels
- Lipid levels, including cholesterol in all patients over 40 years even if there is no indication of risk.

Depression

Mild depression

The treatment involves the following steps:

- Watchful waiting – in mild depression, if the patient does not want treatment or may recover with no intervention, arrange for further assessment, normally within 2 weeks.
- Sleep and anxiety management – consider advice on sleep hygiene and anxiety management.
- Structured and supervised exercise programme – duration between 10 and 12 weeks, up to 3 sessions per week of moderate duration, each session lasting for 45 minutes to 1 hour.
- Guided self-help – this consists of provision of appropriate written materials and limited support over 6–9 weeks, including follow-up from a professional who introduces the programme and reviews the progress and outcome.
- Psychological interventions – the treatment should specifically focus on depression (brief CBT, problem solving therapy and counselling) of 6–8 weeks over 10–12 weeks.
- Where significant co-morbidity exists, consider extending treatment duration or specifically focusing on co-morbid problems.
- Antidepressants – generally not recommended for mild depression, as the risk-to-benefit ratio is poor.

However, consider use of an *antidepressant* for mild depression if:

- It persists after other interventions
- It is associated with medical problems
- It is associated with psychosocial problems
- If a patient with a previous history of moderate or severe depression presents with mild depression.

For patients with depression referred to specialist care, assess patients including their symptom profile, suicide risk, and previous treatment history.

Moderate or severe depression

In moderate depression, offer antidepressant medications to all patients routinely before psychological interventions.

The selection of medications depends on the following factors:

- Severity of the illness
- Previous response to medications
- Response in family members

- Sex of the patient
- Side effect profile
- Toxicity in overdose
- Co-morbidity
- Special features, such as atypical symptoms and psychotic symptoms.

Monitor the risk and review patients periodically.

For patients with a moderate or severe depressive episode, continue antidepressants for *at least 6–9 months after remission.*

- SSRIs are recommended as the *first line drugs* because they are as effective as tricyclic antidepressants and are less likely to be discontinued due to the side effects; tricyclics are more dangerous in overdose (with the exception of lofepramine hydrochloride).
- Consider using a more generic form such as fluoxetine hydrochloride or citalopram as they are associated with fewer discontinuation or withdrawal symptoms.

Once a patient has taken antidepressants for 6 months after remission, review the need for continued antidepressant treatment. This review may include consideration of the number of previous episodes, presence of residual symptoms and concurrent psychosocial difficulties.

- If the patient has not responded well, then check that the drug has been taken regularly and at the prescribed dose.
- If the response is inadequate, and if there are no significant side effects, consider a gradual increase in dose.
- If there is no response after 6–8 weeks, consider switching to another antidepressant.
- But if there has been a partial response, the decision to switch can be postponed for another 6 weeks.
- If the antidepressant has not been effective, or is poorly tolerated, and the decision is made to offer a further course of antidepressants, then switch to another single antidepressant, such as a different SSRI or mirtazapine, reboxetine or a tricyclic antidepressant.
- Inpatient treatment should be considered for people with depression where the patient is at significant risk of suicide or self-harm.

Common causes of hospitalization

- Serious imminent risk of suicide
- Serious long-term high risk of suicide
- Serious risk of harm to others
- Risk of self-neglect
- Severe depressive symptoms

- Severe psychotic symptoms
- Lack of adequate social support
- Severe co-morbid conditions and physical health conditions
- Treatment-resistant cases.

Maintenance therapy

First episode

- The antidepressant treatment should be continued for 6 months to 1 year after remission, particularly if there are residual symptoms.
- The discontinuation should be gradual over a period of *4 to 6 months*.

Recurrent episodes

- Where the depression is chronic or recurrent, assess:
  - Psychosocial stressors
  - Personality factors
  - Significant relationship difficulties.
- In co-morbid depression and anxiety, treat the depression as a priority.
- Continue antidepressant for 2 years for people who have had two or more depressive episodes in the recent past and who have experienced functional impairment during the episodes.
- To prevent relapse, maintain the antidepressant at the same dose at which acute treatment was effective.
- Beyond 2 years, for further continuation of the treatment, re-evaluate patients on maintenance treatment bearing in mind the patients' age, co-morbid conditions and other risk factors.
- If the period between the episodes is less than 3 years, or if it is a severe episode, then prophylactic treatment should be maintained for at least 5 years, as the risk of relapse on stopping medication is 70–90% within 5 years.

Refractory depression

Treatment-resistant depression is defined as failure to respond to adequate courses (dose and duration – maximum BNF dose for at least 6 weeks) of two antidepressants or an antidepressant and ECT.

Treatment strategies

First choice

- Add lithium (aim for a plasma level of 0.4–0.6 mmol/L)

- Add electroconvulsive therapy
- Add high-dose venlafaxine hydrochloride (>200 mg/day)
- Add levothyroxine (20–50 µg/day)
- Add tryptophan
- Fluoxetine hydrochloride and olanzapine.

Venlafaxine hydrochloride may be considered for patients who have failed adequate trials of alternative antidepressants. For patients prescribed with venlafaxine hydrochloride, consider monitoring cardiac function and undertake monitoring of blood pressure for patients on a higher dose.

Consider augmenting an antidepressant with another antidepressant (SSRIs or mirtazapine) and when augmenting one with another, monitor carefully particularly for the symptoms of 'serotonin syndrome'.

Second choice

- Add pindolol (5 mg tds)
- Add dexamethasone (4 mg daily for 4/7 days)
- Add lamotrigine (200 mg/day)
- High-dose tricyclics (imipramine 300 mg/day)
- Add buspirone hydrochloride
- Add monoamine oxidase inhibitors (MAOIs) and tricyclic antidepressant e.g., trimipramine and phenelzine sulfate.

Psychotic depression

- For depression with psychotic features, ECT should be considered as first-line therapy with significant benefit in 80–90% of cases.
- It would be ideal to commence treatment with an antipsychotic agent for a few days before commencing an antidepressant, and use of lowest effective dose of antipsychotics is recommended.
- When combination treatments of antipsychotic and antidepressants are used, careful dose titration is necessary as it may worsen the side effects common to both.
- Following combination treatment, the maintenance often involves a clinically effective antidepressant with the lowest effective antipsychotic dose.

Atypical depression

- Consider prescribing MAOIs such as phenelzine sulfate for patients whose depression has atypical features, on a dose of 15 mg/day increased gradually to 60–90 mg/day, and other MAOIs if necessary; clinically significant advantage in response and remission: Pane et al, 1991 and McGrath et al, 2004.

- All patients receiving phenelzine sulfate require careful monitoring including blood pressure and advice on interaction with other medicines or foodstuffs.
- Alternatives include SSRIs and the noradrenergic reuptake inhibitor (NARI) reboxetine.

Treatment with electroconvulsive therapy

The selection of ECT may be affected by:

- Patient preference
- Previous recovery with ECT
- Previous experience of ineffective and or intolerable medical treatment.

ECT should only be used:

- To achieve rapid and short-term improvement of severe symptoms after an adequate trial of other treatments has proven ineffective
- When the condition is considered to be potentially life-threatening in a severe depressive illness and when the patient is at significant risk of harming themselves or others (potentially life-threatening)
- For a severe depressive episode with severe biological features, such as significant weight loss or loss of appetite
- Where psychotic features are prominent (depressive delusions and/or hallucination)
- In patients who are unable to tolerate the side effects of drug treatment
- When there is a previous history of good response to ECT, if used already
- When there is marked psychomotor retardation
- When there is catatonia or stupor
- When there is treatment-resistant psychosis and mania.

Electroconvulsive therapy is not recommended as a maintenance therapy because its longer-term benefits and risks have not been clearly established (NICE, 2003).

A repeat course of ECT should be considered under the circumstances indicated above only for individuals who have severe depressive illness and who have previously responded well to ECT.

Antidepressants

Side effects

- *Tricyclic antidepressants* (amitriptyline, clomipramine, dothiepin hydrochloride, doxepin hydrochloride, imipramine) – sedation, hypotension, anticholinergic side effects such as dry mouth, constipation, blurred vision, urinary retention, impaired ejaculation, weight gain, ECG changes and arrhythmias

- *Tetracyclic antidepressants* (amoxapine, maprotiline hydrochloride, mianserin hydrochloride) – sedation, drowsiness, dizziness, vivid dreams, dry mouth, constipation, blurred vision, headache, weight gain, tremor
- *Post-synaptic 5-hydroxytryptamine (serotonin) receptor blockers* and reuptake inhibitors (trazodone hydrochloride and nefazodone hydrochloride) – nausea, drowsiness, dizziness, postural hypotension, fatigue, headaches, anticholinergic side effects, bradycardia and elevation of hepatic enzymes
- *Irreversible monoamine oxidase inhibitors* (isocarboxazid, phenelzine sulfate, tranylcypromine sulfate) – drowsiness, insomnia, agitation, dizziness, weakness, fatigue, diarrhoea, weight gain, oedema, postural hypotension and anticholinergic side effects
- *Reversible inhibitor of monoamine oxidase type A* (RIMA; moclobemide) – nausea, headache, dizziness, insomnia, anxiety, restlessness, dry mouth, blurred vision, rash
- *Selective serotonin (5-hydroxytryptamine) reuptake inhibitors* (fluoxetine hydrochloride, paroxetine hydrochloride, sertraline hydrochloride, citalopram, escitalopram)
  - Gastrointestinal side effects – nausea, vomiting, dyspepsia, abdominal pain, diarrhoea
  - CNS side effects – headache, sweating, anxiety, agitation, insomnia
  - Sexual dysfunction
- *Selective noradrenalin reuptake inhibitors (SNRIs)*
  - Venlafaxine hydrochloride – nausea, headaches, dry mouth, dizziness, sweating, somnolence, sexual dysfunction, elevation of blood pressure at higher doses
  - Duloxetine hydrochloride – nausea, dryness of mouth, constipation, diarrhoea, vomiting, decreased appetite, dizziness, somnolence, insomnia
- *Noradrenergic/specific serotonergic antidepressants (NaSSAs)*
  - Mirtazapine – sedation, drowsiness, dizziness, fatigue, increased appetite, weight gain, dry mouth, constipation
  - Reboxetine – insomnia, sweating, dizziness, dry mouth, constipation, tachycardia, urinary hesitancy.

Dosages

Table 7.3 gives the dosage ranges for antidepressants.

Licensed indications

- Amitriptyline – depression, nocturnal enuresis in children
- Clomipramine – depression, phobic and obsessional states
- Dothiepin hydrochloride, doxepin hydrochloride – depression

TABLE **7.3** Dosage ranges for antidepressants

Drug name	Usual daily dose range (mg)
Amitriptyline	100–150
Clomipramine	100–250
Imipramine	100–300
Lofepramine	140–210
Dothiepin hydrochloride	100–225
Doxepin hydrochloride	100–300
Trazodone hydrochloride	150–600
Nefazodone hydrochloride	300–600
Moclobemide	300–600
Phenelzine	45–90
Fluoxetine hydrochloride	20–60
Fluvoxamine hydrochloride	100–300
Citalopram	20–60
Paroxetine hydrochloride	10–50
Sertraline hydrochloride	50–200
Escitalopram	10–20
Venlafaxine hydrochloride	75–375
Mirtazapine	15–45
Reboxetine	8–12
Duloxetine hydrochloride	60–120

- Phenelzine sulfate – depression
- Moclobemide – depression, social phobia
- Trazodone hydrochloride – depression, anxiety
- Nefazodone hydrochloride – depression, anxiety
- Fluoxetine hydrochloride – depression, anxiety, obsessive–compulsive disorder (OCD), bulimia nervosa
- Paroxetine hydrochloride – depression, anxiety, OCD, panic disorder, agoraphobia, social phobia, post-traumatic stress disorder (PTSD), generalized anxiety disorder
- Citalopram – depression, anxiety, panic disorder, agoraphobia
- Escitalopram – depression, anxiety, panic disorder, agoraphobia
- Sertraline hydrochloride – depression, anxiety, OCD
- Fluvoxamine maleate – depression, OCD
- Venlafaxine hydrochloride – depression, generalized anxiety disorder
- Mirtazapine – depression
- Reboxetine – depression
- Duloxetine – depression.

Psychological treatments

The use of the psychological therapies is influenced by the severity of the episode, patient preferences and local availability.

- Cognitive behavioural therapy (CBT) is the psychological treatment of choice and an adequate course involves 16–20 sessions over 6–9 months.
- Also consider interpersonal therapy (IPT) if the patient expresses a preference for it or if you think that they may benefit from it.
- When patients have responded to a course of individual CBT or IPT, consider offering follow-up sessions, typically 2–4 sessions over 12 months.

Cognitive behavioural therapy

Consider CBT:

- If a patient with moderate or severe depression refuses antidepressant treatment
- For patients who have not made an adequate response/have limited or poor response to other interventions for depression
- For patients in whom avoiding the side effects often associated with antidepressants is a clinical priority or personal preference
- For patients who express a preference for psychological treatments.

Cognitive behavioural therapy in depression

In depression, there is pervasive negative view of the self, the world and the future.

The *cognitive* part of CBT includes identifying, evaluating and modifying negative automatic thoughts and dysfunctional beliefs. It involves thought challenging based on Socratic questioning, where the therapist challenges these thoughts constructively and alternative explanations are offered, and it aims to reduce the frequency of negative thoughts.

In depression, CBT aims to restructure the negative cognitions that lead to depression (arbitrary inference, minimization, maximization, selective abstraction, overgeneralization, dichotomous thinking).

The *behavioural* techniques used include:

- Activity scheduling with a plan of action aimed at exploring the relationship between activity and mood
- Mastery and pleasure tasks focusing on self-monitoring of pleasure and a sense of mastery associated with activities
- Graded task assignments breaking goals into achievable subtasks and helping patients to achieve success step-by-step; and specific experiments to test negative prediction.

Research evidence for CBT in depression:

- Cognitive behavioural therapy is as effective as antidepressant medication in mild-to-moderate depression.

- The combination of CBT and antidepressants is not more effective than either treatment alone in mild-to-moderate depression.
- The combination of CBT and antidepressants may be more effective than either treatment alone in severe depression.
- Relapse rates are lower with CBT than with antidepressants following discontinuation of treatment.

Cognitive behavioural therapy combined with antidepressant medication:

- For patients who present initially with severe depression
- For all patients whose depression is treatment-resistant or chronic
- For patients with treatment-resistant moderate depression who have relapsed while taking or after finishing a course of antidepressants.

Consider the combination of antidepressant medication with individual CBT of 16–20 sessions over 6–9 months.

Interpersonal therapy

- It is a time-limited weekly therapy for depressed patients.
- It focuses more on current relationships than on enduring aspects of the personality.
- The therapist takes an active role and explores the connections between the onset of the current symptoms and interpersonal problems in four areas – grief, role transitions, interpersonal role disputes and interpersonal deficits.
- The therapist will concentrate on strategies specific to one of these problem areas.
- The patient is helped to focus on the therapeutic gains and to develop ways of identifying and tackling depressive symptoms.

Bipolar affective disorder

Hypomania, mania and mixed episode (acute treatment phase)

Key points:

- Antipsychotics, sodium valproate and lithium are *antimanic*. The antipsychotics are preferred in highly active or agitated patients with mania.
- The atypical antipsychotics such as olanzapine, risperidone, quetiapine fumarate and aripiprazole have shown 'efficacy as monotherapy' in placebo controlled trials in mania, and atypicals are less likely to produce extrapyramidal symptoms.
- Short-term treatments of mania can be discontinued after full remission of symptoms, which usually lasts for *2–3 months*.
- If the patient has hypomanic or manic symptoms and if the patient is already on an antidepressant, then *taper and discontinue the antidepressant*. Just like the switch from mania to depression, a switch from depression to mania can also occur, which may be a consequence either of the course of the illness or of the treatment.
- If the patient is already on long-term treatment then *optimize* and *continue* the same treatment.
- If the patient is sleep deprived, consider the use of a short-term benzodiazepine. Benzodiazepines are not believed to be antimanic. However, they are used as adjuncts to other agents and may be required when sedation or tranquillization is a priority. The use of benzodiazepines may also reduce the required doses of antipsychotics or other drugs. They should be discontinued after the desired response is established.
- When on maintenance treatment, if mania recurs, then combining an antipsychotic such as olanzapine, risperidone or haloperidol can facilitate the acute treatment response and randomized controlled trials have shown that combinations are superior to lithium or valproate alone.
- Mixed episodes are slower to resolve during treatment than more classic mania.

Depressive episodes

Key points:

- A switch from mania to depression may occur at any time during the course of the illness; it is not established which treatments if any make this more likely to happen.
- If the patient is already on maintenance treatment, then *optimize the therapy* and *continue*.

- Meta analysis has shown that a manic event is 2–3 times more likely to occur during treatment with tricyclic antidepressants than during treatment with SSRIs or placebo.
- Antidepressants are effective for treating depression in bipolar disorder but are used in combination with an agent that will reduce the risk of mania (lithium, or sodium valproate).
- After remission of an acute episode of depression, the discontinuation of antidepressants is currently recommended, but when the risk of a severe depressive episode is high, the antidepressants to which the patient has shown an acute response may be continued long term, either alone or in combination with a drug showing antimanic efficacy.
- Lamotrigine has been shown to have acute efficacy in depression without a risk of inducing switching.
- For manic or mixed states resistant to treatment, or for severe depression electroconvulsive therapy provides an important treatment option.

Rapid cycling bipolar disorder

- Taper and discontinue the antidepressants.
- Identify and treat factors such as substance misuse, hypothyroidism or lithium-induced hypothyroidism that may contribute.
- For initial treatments consider lithium, sodium valproate and lamotrigine – for rapid cycling disorder, sodium valproate is the drug of choice.
- But, if severe, then add an antipsychotic agent (e.g., olanzapine) and also consider benzodiazepines for agitation and insomnia.
- Combinations are often required – evaluate over 6 months or more.
- Generally, antidepressant drugs should be stopped and lithium therapy reduced or sometimes stopped in these patients.

Maintenance therapy

Key points:

- According to NICE guidelines (2006), *lithium, olanzapine or sodium valproate* should be considered for long term treatment of bipolar disorder.
- If the patient has frequent relapses then switching to an *alternative monotherapy* or adding a *second prophylactic agent* (lithium, olanzapine, sodium valproate) should be considered.
- Lithium and olanzapine prevent the relapse of mania, and research evidence suggests that lithium reduces the risk of suicide. Lithium is probably more effective against mania than against depression, with a relative risk reduction of 40% and 23% respectively. Plasma lithium levels of below 0.5 mmol/L are usually too low to be effective and levels over

0.8 mmol/L are often recommended – the highest dose with the minimal side effects should be employed.

- The following conditions predict a relatively poor response to lithium maintenance therapy:
  - Rapid cycling disorders
  - Alcohol and drug misuse
  - Mixed affective states
  - Mood incongruent psychotic features.
- In the prevention of mania, *sodium valproate* has been proved to be as effective as lithium but carbamazepine is less effective than lithium.
- *Lamotrigine* is more effective against depression than mania in long-term treatment, and it has a novel profile in relapse prevention.
- Discontinuation of long-term treatment is not indicated when there is good clinical control of the illness.
- Successful long-term treatment often appears to require combination treatment. Effective prevention of disease progression may require combination therapy from as early in the illness course as possible.
- Antipsychotic agents may often be appropriate for the long-term management of bipolar patients, especially those in whom psychotic features are prominent.
- For those who have frequently recurring episodes and either do not benefit from or do not adhere to oral medication, depot antipsychotic medication can provide long periods of stability.

Mood stabilizers

Side effects

- Lithium – increased thirst, polyuria, polydipsia, bad metallic taste in the mouth, weight gain, nausea, vomiting, abdominal pain, muscular weaknesses, tremors, acne, hypothyroidism
- Carbamazepine – nausea, vomiting, constipation, sedation (dose-related), dizziness, ataxia, diplopia (dose-related), hepatitis, skin rashes, blood dyscrasias
- Sodium valproate – nausea, vomiting, sedation, diarrhoea, ataxia, tremor, hair loss, weight gain, thrombocytopenia, blood dyscrasias, ankle oedema, pancreatitis
- Lamotrigine – rash, ataxia, headache, diplopia, vomiting
- Topiramate – appetite suppression, weight loss, nausea, abdominal pain
- Gabapentin – somnolence, dizziness, ataxia, fatigue.

Dosage

Table 7.4 gives the dosage ranges for mood stabilizers.

TABLE **7.4** Dosage ranges for mood stabilizers

Drug name	Daily dose range recommended (mg)
Lithium carbonate	400–2000
Sodium valproate	500–2500
Carbamazepine	400–1600
Lamotrigine	50–200
Topiramate	25–200

Recommended monitoring for lithium

Pre-lithium work up: FBC, liver function tests, renal function tests, thyroid function tests, ECG, urea and electrolytes.

- Start at 400 mg once daily
- Plasma level:
  - Check after 5–7 days
  - Then check every 5–7 days until the required therapeutic level is reached
  - Once stable, check every 3–6 months
- Check thyroid function and kidney function tests every 6 months.

Recommended monitoring for carbamazepine

- Perform full blood count at baseline and every 2 weeks for the first 2 months and then every 3–6 months.
- Monitor serum carbamazepine levels every 2 weeks for first 2 months and then every 3–6 months.

Recommended monitoring for sodium valproate

- Perform full blood count at baseline and then 6-monthly.
- Check hepatic and renal function at baseline and then 6-monthly.

Alcohol misuse and dependence

Alcohol dependence

Key features of ICD-10 dependence (3 items required) include:

- Compulsion to drink
- Problems in controlling drinking
- Psychological withdrawal symptoms
- Escalating consumption owing to tolerance
- Preoccupation with alcohol to the exclusion of other pursuits
- Increasing time lost to hangovers
- Disregard of evidence that excessive drinking is harmful.

Harmful alcohol use

Harmful use is diagnosed if there is evidence that alcohol is damaging an individual's mental or physical health but the criteria for dependence are not met.

Sensible drinking

- 21 units per week for men.
- 14 units per week for women.
- People over 65 years of age should consume no more than one standard drink per day, 7 standard drinks per week and no more than 2 drinks at any one time.

Pharmacological management

Detoxification

- Treatment of alcohol use disorders typically involves a combination of pharmacotherapy and psychosocial interventions.
- Detoxification is a treatment designed to control both the medical and psychological complications that may occur temporarily after a period of sustained alcohol misuse.
- It usually involves chlordiazepoxide at diminishing doses over 7–10 days with thiamine supplementation.
- The doses of medication should be titrated against withdrawal symptoms.

Outpatient detoxification

- The benzodiazepines are prescribed in alcohol withdrawal in order to control withdrawal symptoms and to reduce the risk of withdrawal seizures.

- Chlordiazepoxide is usually prescribed in a rapidly reducing regimen in order to reduce the development of secondary dependence; it has a lower abuse potential compared with other benzodiazepines.
- Chlordiazepoxide is the drug of choice for most uncomplicated alcohol dependent patients, but if there are doubts about compliance or concerns about drinking at any stage during outpatient detoxification, then the patient should be reviewed and breathalysed before dispensing the next day's supply of the drug.
- Indications for prescribing a reducing regimen:
  - Clinical evidence of alcohol withdrawal features
  - History of alcohol dependence syndrome
  - Consumption of alcohol is greater than 10 units per day over the last 10 days.
- Indication for inpatient detoxification:
  - Symptoms of Wernicke–Korsakoff syndrome
  - Past history of seizures or delirium during withdrawals
  - Acute confusional presentation
  - High risk of suicide
  - History of poly drug misuse
  - Co-morbid mental health illness, e.g., depression, psychosis
  - Lack of stable support in the community, e.g., homelessness
  - Severe malnutrition/severe physical health conditions.

Chlordiazepoxide regimen for moderate and severe dependence

Day 1	20 mg qid
Day 2	15 mg qid
Day 3	10 mg qid
Day 4	5 mg qid
Day 5	5 mg bid

- In severe dependence, even larger doses of chlordiazepoxide may be required and will often require specialist/inpatient treatment.
- For inpatient detoxification, the chlordiazepoxide should be prescribed according to a flexible regimen over the first 24–48 hours with the dosage titrated according to the severity of withdrawal symptoms. This is followed by a 5-day reducing regimen (a typical regimen might be 10–20 mg qid reducing gradually over 5–7 days). This is usually adequate, and longer treatment is rarely helpful or necessary.

Other medications

- Supplementary vitamins – generally, a 4-week course of 100 mg thiamine tds is recommended, but if there are symptoms suggestive of malnourishment or Wernicke–Korsakoff syndrome then parenteral B vitamins are recommended.

- Anticonvulsants – benzodiazepines in sufficient dosage are the most effective anticonvulsant in alcohol withdrawal.
- Antipsychotics – it is generally not advisable to start a new psychotropic at this time as most of the antipsychotics reduce seizure threshold. However, if there are psychotic symptoms, such as delusions or hallucinations, they could be initially managed by increasing the dose of benzodiazepine. The addition of an antipsychotic, such as haloperidol 5–10 mg orally up to 30 mg/day, should be considered if this fails, but given sufficient benzodiazepine cover you should address the concern of a possible reduction in seizure threshold following antipsychotic use.

Maintenance treatments

Aversive drugs:

- Disulfiram:
  - It is an irreversible inhibitor of acetaldehyde dehydrogenase, which can act as an adjunct to therapy and is prescribed once abstinence is achieved.
  - Dose – give a 5-day loading dose of 800 mg/day followed by a maintenance dose of 200 mg or 400 mg on alternate days.
  - Common side effects – headache, halitosis.
  - Rare reports of hepatotoxicity and psychotic reactions have been reported.

Anti-craving drugs:

- Acamprosate calcium:
  - It is believed to act through enhancing γ-aminobutyric acid (GABA) transmission in the brain, and patients taking it report diminished alcohol craving.
  - Dose – 666 mg tds, once abstinence is achieved.
  - Side effects – pruritus, gastrointestinal upset, rash.
- Naltrexone hydrochloride:
  - It antagonizes the effects of endogenous endorphins released by alcohol consumption. It appears to be effective in reducing total alcohol consumed and the number of drinking days.
  - Dose – 50 mg/day, once abstinence is achieved.
  - Side effects – feeling anxious, headache, fatigue, flu-like symptoms, gastrointestinal symptoms, sleep disturbance.

Research evidence

- Research has consistently shown that less intensive treatments are as effective as the more intensive options as there was no difference in outcome measures between both groups (Chick et al, 1988).

- Published reports have consistently failed to identify any significant differences in the outcomes between short and long inpatient detoxification programmes (Miller and Hester, 1986).
- Edwards and Guthrie's trial (Edwards and Guthrie, 1967) reported no significant differences in outcomes between the groups who were randomly assigned to inpatient or intensive outpatient treatment and followed up each month for 1 year and assessed by independent raters.
- Large trials such as Project MATCH (Matching Alcohol Treatment to Clinical Heterogeneity) and UKATT (The United Kingdom Alcohol Treatment Trial) show no significant difference between the various forms of psychosocial treatment.

Psychosocial intervention

Motivational enhancement therapy

Motivationally based treatments concentrate on strategies that focus on the patient's own commitment to change. Motivational enhancement therapy combines counselling in the motivational style with objective feedback.

- It is ideal for use in primary care.
- It is aimed more at the problem substance misuser than the dependent substance misuser.
- It involves several short sessions of a few minutes aimed at increasing internal motivation.

Here, the clients themselves give reasons why they should remain abstinent and draw up a list of problems caused by their alcoholism.

The therapist does not take a directive approach but expresses interest and concern for the patient's problems; uses open-ended questions and reflective listening, which aids the assessment of pros and cons of current behaviour.

Motivational enhancement therapy also encourages the patient's own perceptions of degree of risk, encourages personal responsibility and offers patient's a choice of treatment options.

The principles of motivational interviewing – *FRAMES' formulation:*

F: provide *feedback* on behaviour
R: emphasis on personal *responsibility* for changing behaviour
A: clear *advice* to change
M: A *menu* of alternative options to change behaviour
E: therapeutic *empathy* for the patient as a counselling style
S: facilitation of client *self-efficacy* or optimism.

Cognitive behavioural therapy

Cognitive behavioural therapy is now considered to be the most dominant form of psychological intervention for the treatment of substance misuse. It is particularly helpful in co-morbid conditions, such as anxiety disorders, phobic disorders, PTSD, OCD and depression.

Patients who misuse substances are perceived as not having the skills to cope with other problems and this assumes that alcoholism is a maladaptive habit that becomes a means of coping with difficult situations, unpleasant moods and peer pressure.

The emphasis is placed on *overcoming skill deficits* and increasing the ability to cope with a difficult situation. One of the main benefits of this approach is to help patients to form the coping strategies and resources to fundamentally prevent relapses.

It is typically offered in the following areas:

- Reducing exposure to substances
- Motivating by exploring the positive and negative consequences of continued use
- Self-monitoring to identify situations, settings, or states associated with higher risk for substance use, and coping with negative emotional states
- Recognition of conditioned craving and development of strategies for coping with craving
- Homework assignments
- Identification of thought processes that can increase risk for relapse, and focusing on relapse prevention.

Social skills training is an integral component of CBT. The techniques include assertiveness training, modelling and role playing of skills such as refusal of alcohol and dealing with interpersonal problems. It also focuses on dealing with the social pressure to use drugs, development of supportive networks and development of plans to interrupt a relapse.

Twelve-step facilitation

- Twelve-step facilitation is a form of structured intervention to enhance engagement with Alcoholics Anonymous (AA).
- The objectives include encouraging patients to become members of AA groups and to accept the AA philosophy.
- The basic philosophy of AA is that of reaching out to other alcoholics to help everyone stay sober.
- Group work is central to the approach, and it is grounded in the concept of substance misuse as a spiritual and medical disease.

The outcomes for AA attendees are mixed, as with all forms of treatment for addiction:

- Dropout rates are high and approximately half of those who attend AA leave within 3 months.
- Despite this high dropout rate, for those who remain, the abstinence rate is excellent; the average length of sobriety amongst active members is approximately 6 years.

Brief interventions

Brief interventions are short, focused discussions that usually last less than 15 minutes, which can reduce alcohol consumption in some individuals with hazardous drinking. They are based on motivational interviewing. These are designed to promote awareness of the negative effects of drinking and to motivate change.

Heterogeneous populations of drinkers in primary care favour screening and brief intervention. A brief intervention involves one or more counselling sessions, which include assessment, motivational work, patient education, comparison of the individual's consumption with drinking norms, feedback about the adverse effects of alcohol, contracting by keeping a drink-diary, setting goals and incentives to reduce weekly consumption and the use of written materials and information leaflets.

Counselling

The patients of all specialist services will benefit from access to formal counselling.

Qualified counsellors who are receiving supervision should deliver formal structured counselling, and professionals who provide counselling will need to ensure that the patient's health and social needs are addressed by different team members. It can address the following:

- Problem-solving skills
- Social skills training
- Anger management
- Relaxation training
- Cognitive restructuring
- Relapse prevention.

Marital and family therapies

Examine the role of important others in the addictive process.

Social behaviour and network therapy

These are focused on improving interpersonal functioning and enhancing social support based on the principle that people with serious drinking problems need to develop a social network that supports change. They use techniques adapted from CBT and help the patients to build these networks.

The patients are encouraged to identify and develop alternative reinforcers, such as fulfilling 'social activities with non-drug using others' and 'vocational rehabilitation'. The provision of constructive and purposeful activity to substitute for the social activity should include educational activities such as attending college and general social activities such as attending social clubs and sports activities.

Practical help

Direct practical help with specific tasks such as physical cleaning of the home, securing housing or making child-care arrangements not only provides some relief, but it also creates a framework of trust within which other therapeutic work may then take place.

Supported accommodation

The provision of housing with 24-hour availability of housing support workers can be of particular assistance in the transition from residential rehabilitation to fully independent living.

Opioid misuse and dependence

Opiate withdrawal:

- The withdrawal symptoms appear 6–24 hours after the last dose and typically last 5–7 days, peaking on the second or third day.
- Methadone is longer acting and withdrawal symptoms are much more prolonged with symptoms peaking on the seventh day or so and lasting up to 14 days.

Pharmacological strategies

Methadone hydrochloride

- Currently, methadone is the drug of choice used in opiate detoxification regimens and maintenance.
- Methadone is a long acting synthetic opioid with a long half-life of 24 hours and is suitable for daily dosing.
- It is prescribed as a coloured liquid, available at concentration of 1 mg/mL, but it is unsuitable for parenteral use.
- At doses of more than 80 mg/day it produces near saturation of opioid receptors, minimizing the reward of further consumption.
- Methadone should be initiated according to the severity of withdrawal symptoms – start with 10–20 mg methadone depending on the level of tolerance (low: 10–20 mg; moderate: 25–40 mg).
- Review daily over the first week with dose increments of 5–10 mg/day if indicated; methadone reaches a steady state 5 days after the last dose change.
- Stabilization may take up to 6 weeks to achieve and during this period the patient should be reviewed regularly after the first week, making subsequent increases by 10 mg on each review up to 120 mg.
- In *'rapid reduction regimens'* reduce the dose over 14–21 days using symptomatic drugs as adjuncts.
- *'Slow reduction'* is to be done gradually over a period of 4–6 months reducing by 5–10 mg each fortnight.
- During the process of reduction regimens, make the largest absolute cuts at the beginning and more gradual cuts as the total dose falls.
- Oral methadone is effective in (Wolff et al, 1999):
  – Reducing illicit drug use
  – Reducing injecting
  – Reducing criminal activity
  – Improving physical health
  – Improving social well-being.
- Research evidence has shown that a methadone script reduces street usage, criminality and drug-related mortality.

Buprenorphine (Subutex)

- Buprenorphine is a partial opiate agonist effective in treating opioid dependence.
- It alleviates/prevents opioid withdrawal and craving. It reduces the effects of additional opioid use because of its high receptor affinity.
- It is long-acting and the duration of action is related to the dose administered, and it can be used effectively for shorter-term in-patient detoxifications following the same principles as for methadone.
- Dose increases should be made in increments of 2–4 mg at a time, daily if necessary, up to a maximum daily dose of 32 mg.
- Effective maintenance doses are usually in the range of 12–24 mg daily, which should be achieved within 1–2 weeks of starting buprenorphine.

Lofexidine hydrochloride

- Lofexidine hydrochloride is an alpha-adrenergic agonist given as a 7–10 day treatment course, followed by a gradual withdrawal over 2–4 days.
- Start with 200 µg bid, increased in 200–400 µg steps to a maximum of 2.4 mg/day in 2–4 divided doses.
- Due to risk of postural hypotension blood pressure should be monitored.

Symptomatic medications are used in ameliorating opiate withdrawal symptoms:

- Metoclopramide hydrochloride
  - For treatment of symptoms such as nausea, vomiting
  - 10 mg dose up to maximum of 30 mg/day
- Loperamide hydrochloride
  - For treatment of diarrhoea
  - 4 mg initial dose with 2 mg after each loose stool, maximum dose 16 mg/day
- Ibuprofen
  - For headaches, body aches and muscle pain
  - 400 mg dose up to 1600 mg/day.

Relapse prevention – naltrexone hydrochloride is used as an aid to relapse prevention in previously dependent opiate users who have successfully completed detoxification.

- It should be started at 25 mg and the dose should be increased to 50 mg/day.
- The total dose may be given 3 days per week, which also aids compliance.
- It is also used to facilitate 'rapid detoxification' over 5–7 days in specialist centres.

Harm reduction/minimization

Harm reduction is a kind of strategy taken to reduce the morbidity and mortality for the drug users without necessarily insisting on abstinence from drugs.
A few examples include:

- Advice regarding safe sex
- Advice directed at the use of safer drugs
- Advice directed at safer routes of administration
- Advice regarding safer injecting practice
- Treatment of co-morbid mental or physical health problems
- Engagement with other sources of help
- Prescription of maintenance opiates or benzodiazepines.

General points

- Features of *alcohol* withdrawal:
  - Sweating, coarse tremor, tachycardia, nausea, vomiting, generalized anxiety, psychomotor agitation, occasional visual, tactile or auditory hallucinations
  - Complicated type – 5–15% by grand mal seizures
- Features of *benzodiazepine* withdrawal – anxiety, insomnia, headache, nausea, sweating, agitation, depersonalization, seizures, confusion and delirium
- Features of *opiate* withdrawal – watering eyes and nose, yawning, nausea, vomiting, diarrhoea, tremor, joint pains, muscle cramps, sweating, dilated pupils, tachycardia, hypertension, piloerection (goose-flesh)
- Features of *cannabis* intoxication:
  - Mild euphoria, a sense of enhanced well-being, relaxation, altered time sense, increased appetite, mild tachycardia, variable dysarthria and ataxia.
  - The effects of orally smoked cannabis are slower to begin and more prolonged – if the drug is smoked, the effects of intoxication are apparent within minutes, peaking in 30 minutes and lasting 2–5 hours.
  - Acute harmful effects include mild paranoia, panic attacks and accidents.
  - Chronic harmful effects include anxiety, depression, dysthymia, amotivational syndrome.
  - The drug is not usually associated with physical dependency but it can cause mild withdrawal symptoms including anxiety, insomnia and irritability.
  - Cannabis use is associated with dose-related paranoid ideation, and can precipitate an episode or relapse of schizophrenia.
- Benzodiazepine detoxification

The symptoms of benzodiazepine withdrawal appear within 24 hours of discontinuing a short-acting benzodiazepine, but may be delayed for up to 3 weeks for the longer acting benzodiazepines.

The substitute prescribing in benzodiazepine dependency uses the long-acting diazepam. Convert all benzodiazepine doses to diazepam as per Table 7.5.

The aim is to find the lowest dose that will prevent withdrawal symptoms, and the doses should be divided to prevent over-sedation.

Cut dose by one eighth of total dose each fortnight. For low dose reduce by 2.5 mg fortnightly and for high dose reduce by 5 mg fortnightly.

TABLE 7.5 Benzodiazepines: equivalent dosages (Diazepam – 5 mg)

Drug	Dose (mg)
Lorazepam	0.5 (500 µg)
Nitrazepam	5
Temazepam	10
Chlordiazepoxide	15
Oxazepam	15

Review periodically and if substantial symptoms re-emerge then the dose should be increased temporarily.

Old age (psychosis, depression and dementia)

Old-age psychosis

The prevalence of schizophrenia (early, late and very late onset combined) in the population aged 65 years and above is believed to be about 1%.

Comparison of early-onset and late-onset (onset after 40 years of age) schizophrenia:

- Similarities:
  - Genetic risk
  - Presence and severity of positive symptoms
  - Subtle brain abnormalities revealed by imaging
  - Early psychosocial maladjustments
- Differences – late onset schizophrenia has:
  - Fewer negative symptoms
  - Better response to antipsychotics
  - Better neuropsychological performance.

Characteristic features of very late-onset (after 60 years of age) schizophrenia:

- Lesser likelihood of family history of schizophrenia
- Females more affected than males
- Lesser likelihood of formal thought disorder and affective blunting
- Greater likelihood of visual hallucinations
- Associated social isolation
- Associated sensory deprivation
- Greater risk of developing tardive dyskinesia.

Psychotic symptoms of acute onset are usually seen in delirium secondary to a medical condition, drug misuse and drug-induced psychosis.

Chronic and persistent psychotic symptoms may be due to a primary psychotic disorder such as:

- Chronic schizophrenia
- Late-onset schizophrenia
- Delusional disorders
- Affective disorders
- Psychosis owing to neurodegenerative disorders, such as Alzheimer's disease, vascular dementia, dementia with Lewy bodies or Parkinson's disease
- Chronic medical conditions.

Treatment

- Antipsychotics have been the most commonly used treatment for psychotic symptoms. Their usefulness in treating schizophrenia (both late-onset and very late-onset psychosis) in elderly people is well-established.

- The atypical antipsychotics, which have a better side-effect profile, are considered to be more suitable for elderly people.
- More recently there have been concerns raised regarding the safety of atypical antipsychotics in psychosis due to dementia. The committee on the safety of medicine concluded that olanzapine and risperidone were associated with a two-fold increase in the risk of stroke (a small but significant risk of cerebrovascular events) in elderly patients, especially in people over 80 years, and this restriction has been extended to other atypical antipsychotics.
- In elderly people, age-related bodily changes affect the pharmacokinetics and pharmacodynamics of antipsychotic drugs, which have numerous side effects that can be more persistent and disabling in older people.
- Follow the principle 'START LOW AND GO SLOW'.
- Research literature on the use of conventional antipsychotics suggests significant improvement in psychotic symptoms with the use of haloperidol and trifluoperazine hydrochloride.
- The usefulness of clozapine for treatment-resistant early-onset schizophrenia is well-established, but concerns about the toxicity and the need for monitoring white cell counts due to more frequent occurrence of agranulocytosis has led to limited use in older patients, and it should probably be used in treatment resistance and severe tardive dyskinesia.

The recommended doses of atypical antipsychotics for elderly people are given in Table 7.6, but this should be taken as a guideline and the dosing regimen should be tailored according to the needs of individual patients.

TABLE 7.6 Recommended doses of atypical antipsychotics for elderly people

Drug	Starting dose (mg/day)	Maximum dose (mg/day)
Olanzapine	1–5	5–15
Risperidone	0.25–0.5	2–3
Quetiapine fumarate	12.5–25	100–200
Clozapine	6.25	50–100
Ziprasidone	15–20	80–160

Psychological treatment:

- Psychological treatment involves a novel approach for older people that integrates cognitive behavioural techniques and social skills training. It aims to reduce their cognitive vulnerabilities and improve their ability to cope with stress and to adhere to other forms of treatment.
- Psychosocial intervention, such as a combination of interpersonal and independent skills training together with standard occupational therapy, was associated with improved social functioning and independent living.

Old-age depression

Altered symptoms in late-life depression:

- Reduced complaint of sadness
- Poor subjective memory or dementia-like picture
- Apathy and poor motivation
- Hypochondriasis and somatic concerns
- Late-onset neurotic symptoms, such as late marked anxiety, obsessive–compulsive and hysterical symptoms
- Symptoms such as anorexia, weight loss and reduced energy are difficult to interpret because of co-morbid physical disorders (Koenig et al, 1997).

The most validated screening instrument is the *Geriatric Depression Scale* introduced in 1983.

- Depression in old age is associated with chronicity and a high risk of relapse after recovery.
- Mortality is high in older patients with depression, largely because of concurrent physical disorders.
- The management of depressive disorder is multimodal involving physical, psychological and social modalities, along with multidisciplinary interventions such as psychiatric nurses, social workers, occupational therapists, dieticians, speech and language therapists, physiotherapists and podiatrists.

Treatment

- The treatment for depression in people with dementia, as for depression in other older adults, includes antidepressants, psychosocial interventions or combinations of these and ECT.
- For the older age group, give antidepressant treatment at an age-appropriate dose for a minimum of 6–8 weeks before considering that it is ineffective.
- In the treatment of old-age depression, SSRIs and venlafaxine hydrochloride are to be preferred because of a favourable adverse-effects profile.
- Sertraline hydrochloride has the best evidence for treatment in patients with ischaemic heart disease.
- Sertraline hydrochloride and citalopram have the least potential for drug interactions
- Inappropriate antidiuretic hormone (ADH) secretion may occur as a side effect of all antidepressants, but it is more often linked with SSRIs and the risk factors include increased age, female sex and lower sodium levels.
- Patients with psychotic depression usually require a combined approach with the addition of antipsychotics or ECT.

- Electroconvulsive therapy remains the most effective treatment available for severe depression, particularly in psychotic depression, and the recovery rate is 80%; it is well tolerated even by very elderly people (Tew et al, 1999).
- Electroconvulsive therapy should be avoided in the first 3 months following a stroke or myocardial infarction.
- Elderly patients are more likely to suffer from post-ECT confusion and cognitive impairment, which should be carefully monitored. Unilateral ECT is preferred to bilateral ECT to minimize these side effects.

Treatment-resistant depression:

- If there is a partial response within this period, treatment should be continued for a further 6 weeks as older patients take a longer time to recover, so waiting and supporting the patient may be a reasonable course of action. Consider careful monitoring for side effects and the increased risk of drug interactions.
- Common augmentation strategies include lithium augmentation, combining a tricyclic with an SSRI, combinations such as SSRI and mirtazapine, high-dose venlafaxine hydrochloride.
- Maintenance treatment:
- For a first episode of major depression, the patients should be kept on a continuation treatment of at least 1 year.
- For patients with three or more relapses or recurrences, long-term treatment is usually recommended.
- Once a patient has recovered, there is good evidence that ongoing treatment with a tricyclic, SSRI such as citalopram/sertraline hydrochloride or a combination of medication with a psychological treatment are effective.
- In major depression, the combination of antidepressants with psychotherapy is more effective than either of these treatments alone, especially in relapse prevention.
- Cognitive behavioural therapy is the best established psychological treatment in old-age depression, but interpersonal therapy is also effective in relapse prevention.
- Family therapy has been successfully adapted for use with older adults.
- Psychoeducation has been used with good effect in old-age depression.

Dementia

The assessment of the older patient with mental illness and or cognitive impairment would include the following:

1. Obtaining comprehensive history from the patient, family and carers
2. Full physical and neurological examination

3. Mental state examination including full cognitive assessment
4. Functional assessment (evaluation of ability to perform functions of daily activities)
5. Social assessment (accommodation, benefits, social and leisure activities, financial arrangements, etc.)
6. Assessment of carer's needs.

Therefore, the assessment should focus on *four* important domains:

- Diagnostic assessment
- Functional assessment
- Social assessment
- Carer's assessment

General principles of management of dementias

The management of dementia involves a broad range of key objectives including:

- Diagnosis
- Information
- Treatment of dementia
- Treatment of secondary behavioural and psychological symptoms of dementia (BPSD)
- Organization of a tailored care and support package
- Supporting carers.

Investigations

Baseline blood screening tests:

- Full blood count
- Erythrocyte sedimentation rate (optional)
- Serum B12 and folate level
- Liver function tests
- Urea and electrolytes
- Thyroid function tests
- Calcium and phosphate
- Blood glucose levels
- Serum creatinine.

Further investigations:

- Mid stream urine-culture and sensitivity, urine microscopy, urine dipstick test
- Chest X-ray

- CT of the brain
- ECG
- EEG (only for specific cases)
- Lumbar puncture (only for specific cases)
- MRI of the brain (only for specific cases)
- VDRL (only for specific cases)
- HIV testing (only for specific cases)

Screening tests such as mini mental state examination (MMSE). The MMSE is brief and simple enough for use in routine clinical practice with older patients and it is sufficiently comprehensive that when combined with other clinical measures, it provides a valuable index of dementia severity and staging.

Neuropsychological assessment – a full neuropsychological battery produces a much wider range of scores and examines more domains. The patient will be asked to answer sets of questions to assess their overall intellectual and cognitive function, normalized to the patient's age and baseline and educational level.

The standard neuropsychometric testing battery has the following components:

- Attention
- Abstraction and problem-solving
- Memory
- Orientation
- Motor
- Verbal
- Perceptual/constructional
- Estimated premorbid verbal IQ
- Depression.

These tests should be performed for any patient that the clinician suspects to have cognitive impairment and/or dementia.

- This makes early detection of dementia possible.
- It is particularly helpful in identifying dementia among people with high premorbid functioning.
- It is helpful in discriminating between patients with a dementing illness and those with a focal cerebral disease.

Indications for computed tomography (CT)

- Age less than 60 years
- Sudden onset and rapid deterioration of cognitive symptoms
- Suspicion of a space-occupying lesion or normal pressure hydrocephalus

- Localized neurological signs
- Recent head trauma.

Medical management

- For patients with dementia of Alzheimer's types, *cognitive enhancement* using acetyl cholinesterase inhibitors such as donepezil hydrochloride, rivastigmine and galantamine hydrobromide should be tried.
- Treat behavioural and psychological symptoms of dementia (BPSD) of severe intensity with *antipsychotics*, preferably atypical antipsychotics.
- Treat depressive symptoms with antidepressants preferably *SSRIs, venlafaxine hydrochloride* and *mirtazapine.*
- Treat any other medical illness, and closely liaise with the geriatric team for further advice and management.
- Treat insomnia with sedatives and hypnotics such as zopiclone and zolpidem tartrate.
- For patients with vascular dementia and mixed dementia (Alzheimer-vascular) *general health interventions* include increasing exercise, dietary modification, stopping smoking, managing hypertension and optimizing diabetic control should be tried. Although it is not well-evidenced, *vascular secondary prevention* using aspirin, lipid lowering drugs, antihypertensives and ACE-inhibitors may slow progression.

In older people, the use of psychotropic medications is associated with a number of side effects including:

- Increased risk of falls
- Sedation/drowsiness
- Akathisia
- Parkinsonism
- Tardive dyskinesia
- Risk of cardiac arrhythmias
- Accelerated cognitive decline.

Summary of NICE guidance on acetyl cholinesterase inhibitors:

- The three acetylcholinesterase inhibitors donepezil hydrochloride, rivastigmine and galantamine hydrobromide are recommended as options in the management of patients with Alzheimer's disease of moderate severity only (those with a mini mental state examination [MMSE] of between 10 and 20 points).
- Diagnosis must be made in a specialist clinic and only specialists should initiate treatment.
- Patients who continue on the drug should be reviewed every 6 months by MMSE score and global, functional and behavioural assessment.

- The drug should only be continued while the patient's MMSE score remains at or above 10 points and their global, functional and behavioural condition remains at a level where the drug is considered to be having a worthwhile effect.

Acetylcholinesterases are not only useful to improve cognitive symptoms but research evidence has shown that they are also effective in improving the global outcome, improvement in activities of daily living (ADL) and also in controlling the behavioural and psychological symptoms of dementia.
Common side effects of acetylcholinesterases:

- Donepezil hydrochloride, rivastigmine, galantamine hydrobromide – nausea, vomiting, dizziness, insomnia, diarrhoea
- Memantine hydrochloride – dizziness, confusion, hallucinations.

Note: Memantine hydrochloride is not recommended as a treatment option for patients with moderately severe to severe Alzheimer's disease except as part of well-designed clinical studies.

Roles of other carers

Community psychiatric nurse (CPN)

- To monitor the mental state in the community, monitor compliance with medications, monitor for efficacy and tolerability of medications
- To provide additional support and can coordinate care to involve various agencies.

Occupational therapist (OT)

- To do occupational therapy assessments including home assessments – the functional assessment should focus on encouraging independence with self-care, toilet and feeding, maximizing their mobility and assisting them with communication
- To determine activities of daily living skills and level of functioning, and to ascertain the level of support needed
- To enhance their life skills training, social skills training, problem-solving skills and relaxation techniques; to regain their lost skills and to build up their confidence.

Social services

- To help with community care assessment/assessments of needs – the social management should focus on accommodation, leisure activities, financial matters and legal matters (power of attorney, wills) and also on setting up an appropriate care package including:

- Home care visits (1–4 per day)
- Meals-on-wheels
- Day hospital or day centre attendance
- Respite care in a residential or nursing home
- Long-term placement.

Other groups

- Self-help groups
- Support groups
- Support through day centres/drop-ins
- Supported housing – other placements include independent flats, warden-controlled sheltered accommodation, sheltered-plus accommodation, residential placement, residential EMI placement, nursing home placement
- Voluntary agencies such as the Alzheimer's Society, Age Concern and FISH
- Advocacy services.

Non-pharmacological interventions

Brief psychotherapies:

- Cognitive behavioural therapy
- Interpersonal therapy.

Most of the standard therapies and alternative therapies are usually provided in the day hospital.

- Standard therapies:
  - Behavioural therapy
  - Reminiscence therapy
  - Reality orientation
  - Validation therapy
- Alternative therapies:
  - Activity therapy
  - Art therapy
  - Music therapy
  - Aromatherapy
  - Bright light therapy
  - Multisensory approaches
  - Complementary therapy.

The standard therapies comprise the following:

- *Behavioural therapy* is based on principles of conditioning and learning theory. It is aimed at suppressing or eliminating challenging behaviours and helps to develop more functional behaviours. It requires a detailed period of assessment to identify the ABCs (antecedents, behaviour and consequences); their relationships are made clear to the patient and the interventions are based on an analysis of these findings, changing the context in which the behaviour takes place and using reinforcement strategies that reduce the behaviour. This must be tailored to individual patients' needs with a person-centred approach.

- *Reminiscence therapy* involves helping a person with dementia to relive past experiences, especially those that might be positive and personally significant, for example, weddings, family holidays. It is seen as a way of increasing levels of well-being and providing pleasure and cognitive stimulation. It can be used with individuals or groups, and tends to use activities such as music, art and artefacts to provide stimulation.
- *Reality orientation* therapy aims to help people with memory loss and disorientation by reminding them of facts about themselves and their environment using a range of materials and activities, such as notices, signposts and memory aids. It can be used both with individuals and with groups.
- *Validation therapy* attempts to communicate with individuals with dementia by empathizing with the feelings and meanings hidden beyond their confused speech and behaviour. As a result, the emotional content of what is being said is given more importance than the person's orientation to the present.

Younger people with dementia

Key points:

- There are at least 15,000 people with dementia under 65 years of age in the UK.
- Younger people with dementia make up to 2.2% of all people with dementia (Dementia UK report, 2007).
- Early onset dementia affects more men than women.
- Fronto-temporal dementia is a common cause of dementia in younger people.

The impact of dementia on younger people:

- Isolation
- Emotional burden
- Financial concerns
- Lack of occupation
- Loss of roles
- Relationships and parenthood.

Obsessive–compulsive disorder

- Depression is the most common complication of OCD, and depressive symptoms are common in OCD – as many as a third of OCD patients may fulfil the diagnostic criteria for major depression.
- Many patients suffering from OCD develop co-morbid psychiatric conditions. The co-existing diagnoses in primary OCD are major depressive disorder (65–67%), simple phobia (22%), social phobia (18%) and eating disorder.

Treatment

Most clinicians make a *combined approach* to the treatment of OCD that includes psychological and pharmacological treatment.

- For the successful treatment of OCD, antidepressants with potent effects on the serotonergic neurotransmitter system that appear to have anti-obsessional efficacy should be used.
- OCD does not respond to antidepressants lacking 5-hydroxytryptamine (serotonin) reuptake blocking activity even though these are effective in depression.
- Random controlled trials and placebo-controlled studies have shown that fluoxetine hydrochloride, paroxetine hydrochloride, sertraline hydrochloride and fluvoxamine malate have all shown to be effective in the treatment of OCD.
- The evidence supports the clinical view that higher doses of SSRIs and clomipramine than used in depression are likely to produce a therapeutic effect (Table 7.7).
- On the basis of risk-benefit assessment, the *first choice treatment* should be an *SSRI*. The choice should be made on the safety and tolerability, which favours SSRIs.
- If treatment is initiated at lower dose then patients need to be reviewed for a possible increase in the dose if response is unsatisfactory.
- Most patients treated for OCD may respond within the first few weeks of treatment, but 15–20% of patients respond much later. It is, therefore, important that courses of treatment should be of adequate length.
- Maintenance therapy is warranted, and higher doses may be required than standard antidepressant doses.
- Clomipramine has been shown to be effective in the treatment of OCD in children as well as in adults.
- Compared with clomipramine, the SSRIs have fewer side effects especially anticholinergic side effects (see below), and they have a much-improved safety profile.

- Clomipramine is associated with a substantially elevated level of convulsions reported at 1.5–2% in the higher doses often used in OCD compared with 0.1–0.5% in higher doses of different SSRIs.
- Moreover clomipramine is associated with a higher level of cardiotoxicity that is reflected in the higher rate of deaths from overdose.
- Anxiolytic drugs give some short-term symptomatic relief but should not be prescribed for more than about 3 weeks at a time.
- If anxiolytic treatment is needed for a longer time, small doses of an antipsychotic or tricyclic antidepressants may be used.
- Long-term (up to 12 months) double-blind studies demonstrate an advantage for continuing with medication in patients who have responded to acute treatment.
- There is some evidence that combination treatment is superior to psychological approaches or serotonergic antidepressant treatment when given alone.

TABLE 7.7 Medication with demonstrated efficacy in obsessive-compulsive disorder

Drug	Dose (mg)
Clomipramine	100–300
Fluoxetine hydrochloride	30–60
Fluvoxamine hydrochloride	100–300
Paroxetine hydrochloride	40
Sertraline hydrochloride	50–200

Side effect profiles

- SSRIs – nausea, vomiting, anxiety, transient nervousness, insomnia, sexual problems, gastrointestinal disturbances
- Clomipramine – sedation, orthostatic hypotension, dry mouth, blurred vision, constipation, tachycardia, urinary hesitancy or retention.

Psychological therapy

Cognitive behavioural therapy involves the cognitive part and the behavioural part:

- The *cognitive part* aims to identify and modify maladaptive cognitions such as perfectionist ideals, pathological doubt and magic rituals to prevent catastrophes
- The *behavioural part* involves exposure and response prevention and provision of alternate behaviours. Exposure techniques for obsessions, response prevention for ritualistic behaviour and thought-stopping may help in obsessional ruminations.

Obsessional rituals usually improve with a combination of exposure with response prevention to any environmental cues that increase the symptoms.

Exposure therapy
The patient is exposed to the situations that cause anxiety or catastrophic thoughts, and this is done until the patient feels a marked relief of the anxiety symptoms. One common example for a patient with contamination fears would be to make an exposure with dirty or 'germy' objects. This provokes symptoms of anxiety and may cause severe distress for the patient, but during the course of the therapy the patient will also slowly learn from this experience that no catastrophic event will follow this exposure and so after a period of exposure for few minutes, paradoxically a decrease of anxiety symptoms occurs. This procedure has to be repeated several times with different objects that cause different levels of fear.

Response prevention
The treatment strategy involves exposing the individual to stimuli that trigger anxiety or discomfort, and then having the individual voluntarily refrain from performing his or her ritual or compulsion. Through response-prevention techniques, the aim is to stop and prevent recurrence of the repetitive behaviour. Here again, the patient will experience anxiety and severe discomfort. But as no negative consequences occur, these negative feelings will slowly decrease, and they learn to cope with it with minimal or no anxiety. This helps the patient to face more situations that cause obsessive-compulsive behaviour.

Treatment-resistant obsessive–compulsive disorder

A treatment strategy for treatment-resistant OCD is given in Table 7.8

TABLE **7.8** Treating treatment-resistant obsessive-compulsive disorder

Stage	Strategy	Treatment
1		SSRIs or clomipramine
2	Switch	SSRIs to clomipramine (vice versa)
3	Augment	Lithium, risperidone, quetiapine fumarate, trazodone hydrochloride, pindolol, haloperidol, tryptophan, buspirone hydrochloride
4	Use other treatments	Intravenous clomipramine (rarely used), MAOIs, clonidine, clonazepam
5		Electroconvulsive therapy (rarely used)
6		Psychosurgery: cingulotomy, limbic leucotomy and anterior capsulotomy (rarely used these days)

MAOIs, monoamine oxidase inhibitors; SSRIs, selective serotonin (5-hydroxytryptamine) reuptake inhibitors

Anxiety disorder and phobias

Generalized anxiety disorder

If immediate management of generalized anxiety disorder (GAD) is necessary, any or all of the following should be considered (NICE, 2004)

- Support and information
- Problem-solving
- Benzodiazepines
- Sedative antihistamines
- Self-help.

Acute treatment

Pharmacological

- Antidepressants – SSRIs such as paroxetine hydrochloride, sertraline hydrochloride and escitalopram
- Venlafaxine hydrochloride, imipramine
- Buspirone hydrochloride
- Benzodiazepines such as alprazolam and diazepam, which should not usually be used beyond 2–4 weeks.

Consider an *SSRI as the first-line treatment*; higher doses may be associated with greater response and treatment periods of up to 12 weeks are needed to assess efficacy.

For generalized anxiety disorders, the treatment is focused on predominant anxiety symptoms, but for:

- Depressive symptoms – treat with antidepressants (SSRIs, TCAs, venlafaxine hydrochloride)
- Somatic symptoms – treat with benzodiazepines (lorazepam, diazepam)
- Autonomic symptoms – treat with beta blockers (atenolol, propranalol hydrochloride)
- Psychic symptoms – treat with buspirone hydrochloride.

Psychological

- Cognitive behavioural therapy.

Long-term treatment

- Continue the drug treatment for another 6 months in patients who have shown initial response in the first 12 weeks.
- If the patient responds, then continue treatment for up to a year before trial discontinuation by gradual lowering of dose.

- If symptoms recur, then continue for one more year before considering a second trial discontinuation.
- Treatment of co-morbid psychiatric conditions (depression, alcohol/substance misuse) is highly important and should be addressed in the early stage of treatment.
- Consider cognitive behavioural therapy as it may reduce the relapse rates better than drug treatment.
- If initial treatments fail, then consider combining drug treatments and cognitive behavioural therapy.
- Psychosurgery should be tried if all other interventions fail for severe intractable refractory symptoms.

The interventions that have evidence for the longest duration of effect in descending order are:

1. Psychological therapy (CBT)
2. Pharmacological therapy with antidepressants
3. Self-help.

Panic disorder (with and without agoraphobia)

A combination of pharmacological and psychological approaches is shown to be better than a single approach.

Pharmacological treatment

- Selective serotonin reuptake inhibitors:
  - Paroxetine hydrochloride, fluoxetine hydrochloride, citalopram, sertraline hydrochloride and fluvoxamine malate have all been recommended for the treatment of panic disorders
  - Start at a low dose and increase gradually if panic symptoms increase
- Tricyclic antidepressants:
  - TCAs such as imipramine or clomipramine have been shown to be effective
  - Other possible alternatives include amitriptyline, nortriptyline hydrochloride, desipramine, doxepin hydrochloride
- Others – MAOIs (e.g., phenelzine sulfate), moclobemide, venlafaxine hydrochloride and reboxetine
- Benzodiazepines (e.g., clonazepam, diazepam):
  - Should be used for 1–2 weeks in combination with antidepressants; the rationale behind this is to bring some symptomatic relief until the antidepressant becomes effective
  - Particularly useful for severe, frequent, incapacitating symptoms, but should be used with caution due to potential for abuse, dependence and cognitive impairment in the elderly.

If there is no significant improvement then consider switching to another evidence-based treatment after non-response at 12 weeks (change to different class of agent: SSRI, TCA, MAOI).

Psychological intervention—cognitive behavioural therapy (see below).

Long-term treatment

Consider cognitive therapy with exposure as this may reduce relapse rates better than pharmacological treatment.

Social phobia

Pharmacological treatment

- Selective serotonin reuptake inhibitors – paroxetine hydrochloride, fluoxetine hydrochloride, citalopram, sertraline hydrochloride and fluvoxamine malate have all been recommended as first-line treatments for panic disorders
- Venlafaxine hydrochloride
- Monoamine oxidase inhibitors (e.g., phenelzine hydrochloride), moclobemide
- Anticonvulsants such as gabapentin, pregabalin
- Olanzapine
- Benzodiazepines (e.g., clonazepam).

Long-term treatment

- Continue drug treatment for a further 6 months in patients who are responding at 12 weeks.
- Consider cognitive behavioural therapy with exposure as this may reduce relapse rates better than pharmacological treatment.

Simple phobia

- Use psychological approaches based on exposure techniques as the first-line treatment.
- For patients with distressing symptoms who have not responded to psychological approaches then consider paroxetine hydrochloride or a benzodiazepine.

Cognitive behavioural therapy for anxiety disorders

The cognitive models of anxiety disorders (generalized anxiety disorder, panic disorder, agoraphobias, social phobias) have the following in common:

- Bias in information processing
- Selective attention
- Maladaptive behaviours – safety and avoidance behaviours.

In CBT, the *cognitive* part explores the patient's automatic thoughts and beliefs in a given anxiety-provoking situation and challenges these thoughts with alternative and more plausible explanations.

It involves:

- *Modification of thinking error* (catastrophic misinterpretation in panic disorder, misinterpretation of any situation as threatening in GAD, misinterpretation of social threat in social phobias)
- *Education* about panic attacks/anxiety management
- Teaching about bodily responses associated with anxiety
- Teaching new coping skills and strategies.

The *behavioural* component involves:

- *Anxiety management* – use of relaxation exercises to control anxiety and control of hyperventilation
- Treating *phobic avoidance* by integrated exposure methods, such as modelling, graded exposure and relaxation. The graded task assignments break goals into achievable subtasks and help patients to achieve success step-by-step; they involve specific experiments to test negative prediction
- *Behavioural experiments* usually involve an exercise to induce the symptoms through imagery, role play or hyperventilation followed by asking the patient to drop their safety behaviours such as avoidance, thought control in GAD, avoidance of exercise and controlling breathing in panic disorder
- *Social skills training* – analysis of the skill deficits followed by teaching the skill and a period of practice within and outside the session.

Research evidence

There is strong evidence through a large number of random controlled trials for the efficacy of CBT in depression, agoraphobia, panic disorder, social phobia, specific phobia, obsessive-compulsive disorder and bulimia nervosa.

Post-traumatic stress disorder

Prevention of post-traumatic symptoms

- De-briefing (brief single session interventions) – routine debriefing is not indicated and should not be used in routine practice when delivering services.
- Watchful waiting – where symptoms are mild and have been present for less than 4 weeks after the trauma, watchful waiting, as a way of managing the difficulties presented by people with PTSD, should be considered. A follow-up contact should be arranged within 1 month.
- Trauma-focused CBT (psychological treatment) should be offered to those with severe post-traumatic symptoms lasting 1 month or longer after a traumatic event. It can prevent the emergence of chronic PTSD in individuals with post-traumatic symptoms, and it should be provided on an individual outpatient basis. The treatment should be regular and continuous, usually at least once a week, and the same person should deliver it. The duration of trauma-focused CBT should normally be 8–12 sessions but if initiated earlier within the first month, fewer sessions may be sufficient (NICE, 2005).

Pharmacological treatment

Drug treatment should not be considered as a routine first line treatment.

Other drugs

- Selective serotonin reuptake inhibitors – paroxetine hydrochloride, sertraline hydrochloride, fluoxetine hydrochloride
- Tricyclic antidepressants – amitriptyline, imipramine
- Venlafaxine mirtazapine
- Phenelzine sulfate, lamotrigine.

Higher doses of SSRIs are generally not recommended but individual patients may benefit from higher doses.

In the acute phase of PTSD for the management of sleep disturbance – use a hypnotic medication for short-term use but, if longer-term drug treatment is required, consideration should be given to the use of suitable antidepressants.

Treatment periods of up to 12 weeks are needed to assess efficacy.

Psychological treatment

Trauma-focused individual cognitive behavioural therapy

The therapist aims to explain the traumatic event from the patient's perspective providing information about the normal response to severe stress.

This involves:

- Recall of images of the traumatic events and exposure to situations that are being avoided
- Self-monitoring of symptoms
- Cognitive restructuring through the discussion of evidence for and against the patient's belief systems
- Interpretation of the event and attributions following the event
- Anger management for those who feel angry about the traumatic events and their causes
- Anxiety management and relaxation training.

Other psychological interventions

- Eye movement and desensitization reprocessing (EMDR)
- Supportive therapy/non-directive therapy
- Hypnotherapy
- Psychodynamic therapy.

Eye movement desensitization and reprocessing
This is one of the new interventions used for the treatment of PTSD.

The therapist waves his or her fingers back and forth in front of the patient's eyes, and the patient is asked to track these movements while focusing on a traumatic event. The act of tracking while concentrating seems to allow a different level of processing to occur. The patient is able to review the event more calmly or more completely than before.

It also involves a cognitive behavioural component, where the negative belief about themselves that resulted from the trauma is explored and the patient rates their level of emotions and the extent to which they believe this new belief.

Longer-term treatment

- Continue drug treatment for a further 12 months in patients who are responding at 12 weeks.
- Monitor the efficacy and tolerability regularly during long-term treatment – the best evidence is for SSRIs.

Eating disorders

Anorexia nervosa

Outpatient treatment

Most people with anorexia nervosa can and should be treated in an outpatient setting (NICE recommendations, 2004).

Outpatient management should involve a psychological treatment with physical monitoring provided by a healthcare professional competent to give it and to assess the physical risk of the illness to the patient, and the monitoring should normally continue for at least 6 months (NICE recommendations, 2004).

Inpatient treatment

Inpatient treatment should generally be reserved for situations where:

- Patients have failed to progress with appropriate outpatient therapy
- There is significant risk of suicide
- There is significant risk of severe self harm (NICE recommendations, 2004).

Patients should be admitted to a setting in which skilled refeeding and careful physical monitoring is available in combination with psychosocial interventions.

- The inpatients should follow a structured symptom-focused treatment regimen with the expectation of weight gain to achieve weight restoration.
- The inpatients should receive psychological treatment that focuses on:
  - Eating behaviour
  - Attitudes to weight and shape
  - Wider psychosocial issues.
- In most patients with anorexia nervosa an average weekly weight gain of 0.5–1 kg in inpatient settings and 0.5 kg in outpatient settings should be the aim of treatment. This requires approximately 3500 to 7000 extra calories per week.
- Following weight restoration, the patient should be offered outpatient psychological treatment, and typically this outpatient treatment and physical monitoring following inpatient weight restoration should continue for at least 12 months.
- No drugs have been shown to be of specific benefit in the treatment of anorexia nervosa; therefore, the main treatment approach must be psychological in nature including:
  - Cognitive behavioural therapy
  - Interpersonal therapy

- Focal psychodynamic therapy
- Family interventions focused explicitly on eating disorders for children and adolescents (NICE recommendations, 2004).
- The therapist needs to be flexible and willing to attend to the physical as well as the psychological issues presented by the patient.
- Therapists from the psychodynamic tradition may need to be more active than usual, but those with a cognitive behavioural approach may need to spend more time than usual exploring the complexities of their patients' attitudes to their illness.
- Unfortunately, no one approach has been demonstrated to be convincingly better than any other (Fairburn, 2005).
- For adolescent patients, there is a clear consensus that it is helpful for clinicians to involve the family in treatment (Russell et al, 1987), which leads to the recommendation of conjoint family therapy involving the patient, family and therapist meeting together, or family counselling in which the clinician meets separately with the patient and her family.

A *combined approach* is beneficial compared with an individual approach and has a more favourable outcome.

- *Education* – nutritional education to challenge overvalued ideas, self-help manuals
- *Pharmacological* – fluoxetine hydrochloride, tricyclic antidepressants
- *Psychological* – family therapy, individual psychodynamic therapy, cognitive behavioural therapy.

Inpatient treatment will also be considered if:

- Body mass index (BMI) is less than 13.5
- There is extremely rapid or excessive weight loss
- Severe physical health complications occur such as electrolyte imbalance, hypotension, bradycardia or hypothermia
- There is significant deterioration in mental health.

The goals of inpatient therapy should be fully discussed with the patient and the family:

- Addressing physical and psychiatric complications
- Development of a healthy meal plan
- Addressing underlying conflicts, such as low self-esteem and planning new coping strategies
- Enhancing communication skills (Semple et al, 2005).

Physical complications

- Endocrine changes

- – Growth hormone levels raised
- – Cortisol (positive DST) level raised
- – Gonadotrophin levels decreased
- – Oestrogen level decreased
- – Testosterone level decreased
- – T3 levels decreased
- – Amenorrhoea/loss of libido
- Metabolic abnormalities
  - – Dehydration, hypoglycaemia and impaired glucose tolerance, hyper-cholesterolaemia
  - – Deranged liver function tests, hypokalemia, hypoproteinemia
  - – Plasma amylase (raised), lowered calcium, magnesium and phosphate levels
- Haematological problems
  - – Normochromic, normocytic or iron-deficient anaemia
  - – Leucopoenia, with a relative lymphocytosis, low erythrocyte sedimentation rate (ESR), hypocellular marrow
- Cardiovascular problems
  - – Peripheral oedema, congestive cardiac failure, bradycardia, hypotension
  - – Decreased heart size, QT prolongation
- Gastrointestinal problems
  - – Swollen salivary glands, dental caries, erosion of enamel (vomiting)
  - – Delayed gastric emptying, acute gastric dilations (bulimic episodes, vigorous refeeding, constipation), acute pancreatitis
- Renal problems
  - – Acute/chronic renal failure, hypokalemic nephropathy
  - – Proteinuria and reduced glomerular filtration rate (GFR), raised urea and creatinine
- Musculoskeletal problems
  - – Osteoporosis, pathological myopathy, proximal myopathy, stunted growth
  - – Muscle cramps.

Bulimia nervosa

Primary care – self-help programme
   Six steps in self-help manual:

1. Monitoring
2. Establishing a meal plan
3. Learning to intervene
4. Problem-solving

5. Eliminating dieting
6. Changing your mind.

Combined approaches improve outcomes.

Outpatient treatment

- Antidepressant treatment – SSRIs (especially fluoxetine hydrochloride at a higher dose of 60 mg) are the drugs of first choice for the treatment of bulimia nervosa in terms of acceptability, tolerability and reduction of symptoms. Long-term treatment for more than 1 year is usually necessary.
- Group therapy – guided self-help (bibliotherapy) is useful with education and support, often in a group setting. The treatment usually takes about 4 months and requires 8–10 meetings with the facilitator, appropriate for patients in primary care settings.

Specialist unit

- Inpatient care – recommended in the following situations:
    - If the patient is at high risk of suicide or severe self-harm
    - If there are severe physical health problems
    - In refractory cases
    - If the patient is pregnant and the risk of abortion is high
- Cognitive behavioural therapy – course of treatment should be for 16–20 sessions over 4–5 months. The preferred psychotherapeutic treatment for bulimia nervosa is CBT, which aims to normalize eating habits, and cognitive techniques are designed to modify the excessive concerns about shape and weight. CBT is also helpful to bring improvement in mood symptoms; social functioning and self-esteem also improve with well-maintained effects and low relapse rates
- Interpersonal psychotherapy – may be effective in the long-term but acts less quickly.

Specific physical health problems associated with bulimia nervosa

- Electrolyte disturbances – hyponatraemia, hypokalaemia
- Vomiting – metabolic alkalosis
- Dental erosion
- Constipation
- Oesophageal erosions
- Gastric and duodenal ulcers
- Pancreatitis
- Leucopoenia and lymphocytosis
- Arrhythmias and cardiac failure.

Borderline personality disorder

Indicators for admission of patients with borderline PD

1. Crisis intervention, to reduce risk of suicide or violence to others
2. Co-morbid psychiatric illness such as brief psychotic episode or depression
3. To review the diagnosis, treatment plan and perform full risk assessment
4. To stabilize existing medication regimens

Treatment strategies

Drug treatments are normally considered as an *adjunctive* rather than a primary treatment for borderline PD. However patients with several symptoms of borderline PD such as affective instability, impulsivity, suicidal and self-harming behaviour and transient stress related psychotic symptoms might respond to drug treatments.

However, prior to prescribing, the use and effects of medications need to be discussed with the patient, the target symptoms should be clearly identified, an agreement should be made about the duration of treatment and a method to monitor its effect on symptoms established.

The effects of psychotropic medications are modest, which should be explained to the patient and family.

- For *affective dysregulation symptoms* characterized by depressed mood, mood lability, rejection sensitivity, inappropriate intense anger, the initial treatment is with high doses of SSRIs. If this proves to be ineffective, then switch to antidepressants that target multiple neurotransmitter systems such as venlafaxine.
- For *impulse control disorder* characterized by impulsive aggressive episodes, self-mutilating behaviour or self-damaging behaviour such as substance misuse, reckless spending etc., SSRIs can also be helpful and could be augmented by the addition of lithium, sodium valproate or low dosage neuroleptics.
- Up to 50% of people with borderline PD may also have a *bipolar spectrum* disorder and mood stabilizers such as valproate semi sodium and lamotrigine have both been found to reduce anger, aggression and impulsivity in open studies.
- If prominent stress related *psychotic symptoms* are present then atypical antipsychotics such as olanzapine and risperidone can be added. Clozapine has also been used in patients exhibiting self-mutilation in the context of psychosis.

Although the benefits of medications in borderline PD remain modest, a number of studies have reported improvements when medication is associated with psychological approaches including psychodynamic, cognitive behavioural and dialectical behavioural therapies, although such treatments are more likely to be used after the patient has been discharged from in-patient care (American Psychiatric Association, 2002)

Dialectical behavioural therapy

- Marsha Linehan introduced dialectical behavioural therapy (DBT) as a treatment for borderline PD in 1991.
- The length of treatment is usually about 12 months but it can be extended.
- The different phases of treatment would include assessment phase and stages 1, 2 and 3.

DBT is split into two basic components:

- *DBT skills group* – this occurs weekly; it is highly skills orientated and the aim is to improve the patient's capabilities through learning new skills. The group therapy focuses on distress tolerance skills, development of interpersonal skills and emotional regulation skills.
- *Mindfulness training* focusing on the 'here and now' and which is based on *meditation* techniques plays a key role as part of DBT.

The three stages are:

- Stage 1, *individual therapy* – this focuses on a detailed cognitive behav-ioural approach to self-harm behaviours. It involves recording of episodes of DSH and exploration of internal and external antecedents. A problem-solving approach is adopted, which helps to balance empathy and concern with the notion that the individual is ultimately responsible for his or her own behaviour. The individual sessions are also held weekly and the aim is to help clients to apply their skills training.
- Stage 2 – patients are helped to process previous trauma, explore the underlying historical causes of dysfunction and focus on emotional pro-cessing of previous traumatic experiences.
- Stage 3 – the focus is on developing self-esteem and establishes realistic future goals.

One of the unique features of DBT is that when difficulties arise, patients may contact the therapist by *telephone* between sessions to help them apply skills.

Research evidence and RCTs have shown that DBT helps to reduce delib-erate self harm behaviour and reduces hospital admission for patients with borderline PD.

Principles of management of patients with borderline personality disorder in inpatient units (Gabbard et al, 2000)

- Maintain flexibility

- Establish conditions to make the patient safe
- Tolerate intense anger, aggression and hate
- Promote reflection
- Set necessary limits
- Establish and maintain the therapeutic alliance
- Avoid splitting between psychotherapy and pharmacotherapy
- Avoid or understand splitting between different members of staff either in hospital or in community
- Maintain counter-transference feelings.

Discharge planning

- In the CPA meeting clear boundaries, expectations and responsibilities, crisis and contingency plans should be discussed.
- Effective communication and sharing of ideas should be established between inpatient and community teams.

8

Prognosis

- At the end of each clinical assessment, it is important to review both good and poor prognostic factors, both in terms of the immediate outcome concerning the particular episode and the longer term.

Consider:

- Immediate/short term – good and poor prognostic factors
- Long term – good and poor prognostic factors.

Schizophrenia

Good prognostic factors

- Acute or abrupt onset
- Late onset of the illness
- Short duration
- Presence of precipitating stressor
- Female sex
- First episode of the illness
- Presence of family history of mood disorder
- Good social support
- No history of co-morbid substance misuse
- Good premorbid personality traits
- Presence of mood symptoms
- Presence of positive symptoms
- Presence of good insight
- Good compliance with treatment.

Poor prognostic factors

- Insidious onset
- Early age of onset
- Chronic course of the illness

- Absence of precipitating stressor
- Male sex
- Past history of similar episodes
- Family history of schizophrenia
- Poor social support
- Co-morbid substance misuse
- Poor premorbid adjustment
- Absence of mood symptoms
- Presence of negative symptoms
- Lack of insight
- Poor compliance with treatment
- Institutionalization or long-term hospitalization.
- Low premorbid IQ
- Longer duration of untreated illness.

Best predictors of relapse in the short term

- Non-compliance with medications
- High expressed emotion
- Stressful life events (3 weeks prior to relapse).

Schizoaffective disorder

Depressive symptoms are more likely to run a chronic course compared with manic presentation. The good/poor prognostic factors are the same as those for schizophrenia.

Mood disorders

Good prognostic factors

- Acute or abrupt onset
- Earlier age of onset
- Typical clinical features
- Severe depression
- Well-adjusted premorbid personality
- Good response to treatment.

Poor prognostic factors

- Insidious onset
- Later age of onset (elderly patient)
- Time to initial treatment

- Long duration of index episode
- Severe index episode
- High number of previous episodes
- Family history of affective disorder
- Recent major stressful life events
- Co-morbid anxiety
- Co-morbid substance misuse
- Co-morbid physical disease
- Co-morbid personality disorders
- Premorbid neuroticism
- Underlying dysthymia
- Unfavourable early environment
- Mood-incongruent psychotic features
- Poor drug compliance
- Marked hypochondriacal features
- Double depression.

Clues to possible bipolarity for patients with unipolar depression

- Early age of onset
- Recurrent episodes of depression, usually of short duration
- History of bipolar disorders in relatives
- Presence of psychotic features
- Post partum onset
- Poor or short-lived response to antidepressants
- Manic symptoms induced by antidepressants or electroconvulsive therapy
- Atypical depressive features, such as weight gain or hyperphagia.

The prognosis for bipolar disorder is worse than for unipolar disorder, both in terms of recurrences and recovery. When compared with those with unipolar disorder, those with bipolar disorder showed more frequent but shorter episodes. Late onset of affective illness was associated with chronicity, and recovery was more frequent among unipolar than among bipolar patients.

Follow-up studies over 25 years show a definite recovery in:

- 25% of depressed patients
- 16% of bipolar patients.

Drug and alcohol misuse

Good prognostic factors

- Patient motivated to change
- Patient accepting of appropriate treatment goal
- Supportive family or relationships

- Patient in employment
- 'Alcoholics Anonymous' (AA) involvement
- Treatable co-morbid illness, such as social phobia or anxiety.

Poor prognostic factors

- Ambivalence to change
- Homelessness
- Unstable accommodation
- Repeated treatment failures
- Cognitive impairment
- Drinking embedded into lifestyle.

Obsessive–compulsive disorder

Good prognostic factors

- Good premorbid social and occupational functioning
- Clear precipitating event
- Episodic symptoms.

Poor prognostic factors

- Early onset
- Longer duration of illness
- Co-morbid depression
- Bizarre compulsions
- Giving in to compulsions
- Overvalued ideas or delusional beliefs
- History of personality disorder (schizotypal PD).

Eating disorders

Anorexia nervosa

Good prognostic factors

- Younger age of onset
- No bulimic episodes
- Fewer previous hospitalizations.

Poor prognostic factors

- Male sex
- Late age of onset

- Duration of the illness (chronic)
- Excessive weight loss
- Bulimic features (vomiting/purging)
- Poor parental relationships
- Poor childhood maladjustments/premorbid personality traits
- Anxiety when eating with others
- Poor social support
- Extreme treatment avoidance – compulsory treatment required.

Bulimia nervosa

Poor prognostic factors

- Severe personality disorder
- Low self-esteem.

Alzheimer's dementia

Poor prognostic factors

- Male sex
- Onset before 65 years of age
- Prominent behavioural problems
- Presence of mood symptoms, such as depression
- Parietal lobe damage
- Severe focal cognitive deficits, such as apraxia
- Absence of misidentification syndromes.

9

Tasks for mini assessed clinical encounters (mini-ACEs)

Eliciting symptoms of depression and suicidality

- How are you feeling in yourself?
- How bad has it been?
- Have you cried at all?
- If I were to ask you to rate your mood, on a scale of 0 to 10 where 0 is the rock bottom of how you feel, and 10 is the best of your spirits, where would you place your mood over the last couple of weeks?
- Can you enjoy anything?
- What are the things that you find enjoyable/interesting?
- Is the level of enjoyment the same as before?
- Have you lost enjoyment for things you used to enjoy?
- How have you been in your energy levels these days?
- Have you been feeling drained of energy lately?
- Have you wanted to stay away from other people?
- How do you spend your day?

Biological symptoms

- How has your sleep been recently?
- Do you need less sleep than usual?
- Have you had any trouble getting off to sleep?
- Do you wake early in the morning?
- Is your depression/mood worse at any particular time of day?
- What is the best time/worst time of the day for you?
- What has your appetite been like recently?
- Have you lost any weight lately?
- Has there been any change in your interest in sex?

Cognitive symptoms

- How has your concentration been lately?
- How has been your memory been recently?
- How confident do you feel in yourself?
- How do you describe your self-esteem to be?

Eliciting suicidal intent and negative thoughts

- Have you felt that life wasn't worth living?
- How do you see the future?
- Do you feel inferior to others or even worthless?
- Do you feel hopeless about yourself? Has life seemed quite hopeless?
- Do you feel helpless?
- Do you feel that life is a burden?
- Do you wish yourself dead? Why do you feel this way?
- Have you ever felt like 'ending it all'?
- Did you actually try?
- How do you feel about it now?
- Would you do anything to harm yourself or to hurt yourself?
- Have you got any plans to end your life? What plans?

Eliciting feelings of guilt

- Do you feel that you've done something wrong?
- Do you feel guilty about things?
- Do you tend to blame yourself at all?
- Do you tend to blame anyone else for your problems?
- Do you have any regrets?
- Do you feel that you've committed a crime, or sinned greatly or deserve punishment?

Duration, course, effects, coping

- How long have you been feeling like this?
- What do you think might have caused this?
- How is it affecting your life?
- How do you manage to cope?
- Do you get any help?

Eliciting manic/hypomanic symptoms

- How are you feeling in yourself?
- Have you sometimes felt unusually/particularly cheerful and on top of the world, without any reason?

- If I were to ask you to rate your mood, on a scale of 1 to 10, how would you rate your mood now?
- Have you felt so irritable recently that you shouted at people or started fights or arguments?
- How is your energy level?
- Do you find yourself extremely active but not getting tired?
- Have you felt particularly full of energy lately (or) full of exciting ideas?
- Have you felt that you were much more active or did many more things than usual?

Biological symptoms

- How are you sleeping?
- Do you need less sleep than usual and found you did not really miss it?
- How has your appetite been like recently?
- Have you lost /gained any weight?
- How is the sexual side of your relationship?
- Have you been more interested in sex recently than usual?

Cognitive symptoms

- How has your concentration been like recently?
- What is your thinking like at the moment?
- Are you able to think clearly?
- Do your thoughts drift off so that you do not take things in?
- Do you find that many thoughts race through your mind and you could not slow your mind down?

Over-optimistic ideation and grandiose ideas

- How confident do you feel in yourself?
- Do you feel much more self-confident than usual?
- How do you describe your self-esteem to be?
- How do you see yourself compared to others?
- Are you specially chosen in any way?
- Do you have any special powers or abilities quite out of the ordinary? Do you have any special gifts or talents? If so, what are they?
- Is there a special mission to your life?
- Are you a prominent person or related to someone prominent like royalty?
- Are you very rich or famous?
- Have you felt especially healthy?
- Have you developed new interests lately?

- Have you been buying interesting things recently?
- Tell me about your plans for the future? Do you have any special plans?

Clarification

- If the patient harbours grandiose delusions, then pick up the clues from what the patient says to you.
- Invite the patient to elaborate further on a positive response. Always probe for further elaboration of the beliefs and seek examples.
- Always try to assess the degree of conviction, explanation, effects and coping.

Tendency to engage in behaviour that could have serious consequences

- Has there ever been a period of time when you were not your usual self and you did things that were unusual for you like spending too much money that got you into trouble?
- Has there ever been a period of time when you were not your usual self and you did things that other people might have thought were excessive, foolish or risky?

Explore in detail about the symptom history, mode of onset, duration, progress, precipitating factors and associated problems.

Duration, course, effects, coping

- How long have you been feeling this way?
- What do you think might have caused this?
- How is it affecting your life?
- How do you manage to cope?
- Do you get any help?

Rule out co-morbidity such as:

- Depression
- Psychotic symptoms
- Coping mechanisms i.e. Drug and alcohol misuse.

Eliciting history of hallucinations

Auditory hallucinations

- I understand that recently you have been hearing voices when there is no one around you and nothing else to explain it. Can you tell me more about it?

OR

- I should like to ask you a routine question, which we ask of everybody. Do you ever seem to hear voices or noises when there is no one about and nothing else to explain it? If the patient says 'yes' explore more about it.

Elementary hallucinations

- Do you hear noises like tapping or music?
- What is it like?
- Can you make out the words?
- Does it sound like muttering or whispering?

Second person auditory hallucinations

- Do you hear voices?
- How many voices do you hear?
- Can you give me an example?
- Do they speak directly to you?
- Do they tell you what to do?
- Can you carry on two-way conversation with the voices?
- Do you hear your name being called?
- Who is it you are talking to?
- What is the explanation?

Third person hallucinations

- Do you hear several voices talking about you?

OR

- Do they refer to you as 'he' or 'she' like a third person?
- What do they say?
- Do you hear voices like a running commentary instructing you to do things?
- Do they seem to comment on what you are thinking, reading or doing?
- Do the voices belong to men, women or children?
- Can you recognize those voices?
- If you recognize them, whose voices are they?

Confirm whether they are true hallucinations

- Where do these voices come from?
- Do you hear them in your mind or in your ears?
- Do the voices come from inside or outside your head?

- Do you hear them as clearly as you hear me?
- Can you start or stop them?
- Do you feel that they are real or do you feel that they are just voices?

Hypnagogic/hypnapompic hallucination

- When did this occur? Were you fully awake when you heard these voices?
- Do these voices disturb your sleep?
- Do you hear them more at any particular time like when you go to bed or when you wake up?

Visual hallucination

- Have you seen things that other people can't see?
  – With your eyes or in your mind?
- What did you see?
- Were you half asleep at that time?
- Has it occurred when you are fully awake?
- Did you realize that you were fully awake?
- How do you explain it?

Olfactory hallucination

- Is there anything unusual about the way things feel, taste or smell?
- Do you sometimes notice strange smells that other people don't notice?

Gustatory hallucination

- Have you noticed that food or drink seems to have an unusual taste recently?

Tactile hallucination

- Have you had any strange or unusual feelings in your body?
- Do you ever feel that someone is touching you, but when you look there is nobody there?

Somatic hallucination

- Some people have funny sensations on the body, for example, insects crawling or electricity passing or muscles being stretched or squeezed – have you had any such experiences?
- How do you explain it?

Duration, course, effects, coping

- How long have you experienced them?
- How often do you experience them?
- What do you think might have caused this?
- Why do you think they are happening to you?
- How is it affecting your life?
- How do you manage to cope?
- Do you get any help?

Eliciting details of delusions and abnormal experiences

Start with open questions and then proceed to closed questions.

- Have you experienced anything strange, bizarre or unusual? Or perhaps something that has puzzled you?
- Does anything interfere with your thoughts in any way?

Delusions of persecution

- How well have you been getting on with people?
- Do you ever feel uncomfortable as if people are watching you or talking about you behind your back?
- Is anyone trying to harm, or interfere with you or make your life miserable?
- Is anyone deliberately trying to poison you or to kill you?
- Is there any organization, such as the Mafia, behind it?

Delusions of reference

- Do people seem to drop hints about you or say things with a special meaning?
- Does everyone seem to gossip about you? Or spy on you?
- Do you see any messages for yourself/reference to yourself on TV or radio or in the newspapers?
- Do things seem to be specially arranged?

Delusions of control

- Is anyone trying to control you?
- Do you feel that you are under the control of a person or force other than yourself?
- Do you feel as if you are a robot or zombie with no will of your own?

- Do they force you to think, say or do things?
- Do they change the way you feel in yourself?

Delusions of grandiosity

- How do you see yourself compared with others?
- Is there something out of the ordinary about you?
- Do you have any special power or abilities?
- Are you specially chosen in any way?
- Is there a special mission to your life?
- Are you a prominent person or related to someone prominent like royalty?
- Are you very rich or famous?
- What about special plans?

Delusions of guilt

- Do you feel you have done something wrong?
- Do you have any regrets?
- Do you have guilt feelings as if you have committed a crime or a sin?
- Do you feel you deserve punishment?

Nihilistic delusions

- How do you see the future?
- Do you feel something terrible has happened or will happen to you?
- Do you feel that you have died?
- Has part of your body died or been removed?
- Enquire about being doomed, being a pauper, intestines being blocked, etc.

Religious delusions

- Are you especially close to God or Christ?
- Can God communicate with you?

Hypochondriacal delusions

- How is your health?
- Are you concerned that you might have a serious illness?

Delusions of jealousy

- Can you tell me about your relationship?
- Do you feel that your partner reciprocates your loyalty?

If the patient says 'yes' to any of the delusions, then pick up the clues from what the patient says to you.

Assess the degree of conviction, explanation, effects and coping. Also assess their onset (primary/secondary) and their fixity (partial/complete).

Conviction, explanation, effects, coping

- What do you think is causing these experiences?
- Who do you think is causing them?
- Why do they do so?
- And how do they do that?
- How would you explain them?
- Ask how he/she copes with these thoughts, what he/she has done and what he/she intends to do about them.

Onset and fixity

Always check whether the delusion is:

- Primary or secondary
  - How did it come into your mind that this was the explanation?
  - Did it happen suddenly or out of the blue?
  - How did it begin?
- Partial or full
  - Even when you seemed to be most convinced, do you really feel in the back of your mind that it might well not be true, that it might be your imagination?

OR

  - Do you ever worry that all of this may be due to your mind playing tricks?

Assessing first rank symptoms of schizophrenia

Schneider's first rank symptoms

- Hearing thoughts spoken aloud
- Third person auditory hallucinations
- Running commentary hallucinations
- Thought withdrawal
- Thought insertion
- Thought broadcasting
- Made volition

- Made feelings
- Made impulses
- Somatic passivity
- Delusional perception.

Open question

- I gather that you have been through a lot of stress and strain recently. When under stress sometimes people have certain unusual experiences. By unusual experience I mean, for example, hearing noises or voices when there is no one around. Have you had any such experiences?

If the patient says 'Yes' explore more about the voices:

- Can you tell me more about the voices?

Third person auditory hallucinations

- Do the voices speak among themselves?
- Do you hear several voices talking about you?
- Do they refer to you as 'he' (or 'she'), as a third person?
- What do they say?

Running commentary hallucinations

- Do they seem to comment on what you are thinking, reading or doing?

OR

- Do you hear voices like a running commentary instructing you to do things?

Hearing thoughts spoken aloud

- Can you hear what you are thinking?
- Do the voices repeat your thoughts?
- Do you ever seem to hear your own thoughts echoed or repeated?
- What is it like?
- How do you explain it?
- Where does it come from?

Thought alienation phenomenon (open question)

- Are you able to think clearly?
- Is there any interference with your thoughts?

Thought broadcasting

- Do you feel that your thoughts are private or are they accessible to others in any way?
- Are your thoughts broadcast, so that other people know what you are thinking?
- Can other people read your mind?
- How do you know?
- How do you explain it?

Thought insertion

- Are thoughts put into your head that you know are not your own?
- How do you know they are not your own?
- Where do they come from?

Thought withdrawal

- Do your thoughts ever seem to be taken from your head, as though some external person or force were removing them?

OR

- Do your thoughts disappear or seem to be taken out of your head?
- Could someone take your thoughts out of your head?
- Would that leave your mind empty or blank?
- Can you give an example?
- How do you explain it?

Passivity of feelings or actions

- Are you always in control of what you feel and do?
- Do you feel in control of your thoughts, actions and will?
- Is there something or someone trying to control you?
- Do you feel under the control of some force or power other than yourself, as though you are a robot or a zombie without a will of your own?
- Does this force make your movements for you without you willing it?
- Does this force or power force its feelings onto you against your will?
- Does this force have any other influence on your body?

Somatic passivity

- Are you possessed?
- What does that feel like? How does this force influence you?
- Does it ever make your movements for you?

- Does this force have any other influence on your body?
- Can you describe it for me?

Delusional perception

- Did you at any time realize that things happening around you have a special meaning for you? Can you please give me an example?
- Can you explain that? What happened exactly? Has a sudden explanation occurred out of the blue to you?

Effects, coping

- What do you think is causing these experiences?
- Who do you think is causing them?
- Why do they do so? And how do they do that?
- How would you explain them?
- Could it be your imagination?
- How long have you had these experiences?
- How do they affect you?
- How do they make you feel?
- How do you cope with them?
- What do you intend to do about them?

Eliciting alcohol history

Current usage, longitudinal history and features of dependence syndrome.

Edwards and Gross' alcohol dependence syndrome (1976)

- Subjective awareness of the compulsion to drink
- Increased tolerance
- Withdrawal symptoms
- Salience of drinking behaviour
- Reinstatement after abstinence
- Narrowing of drinking repertoire
- Relief drinking.

Questions

- Current usage in a typical day/week
  - Do you drink alcohol at all?
  - What do you usually drink?

- How often do you have a drink?
- Describe a typical day for me. Could you describe any pattern?
- How many drinks do you have on a typical day of drinking?
- What sort of effect does alcohol have on you?
- Longitudinal history
  - When did it all start?
  - What was the first drink?
  - With whom did you have the first drink?
  - Was it of your own free will (or) peer pressure?
  - How did you progress to the current level?
    a. Started drinking occasionally (social drink)
    b. Regular weekend drinking
  - How much would you drink at the weekend?
  - Do you drink during the week?
    a. Regular evening drinking
    b. Regular lunchtime drinking
    c. Early morning drinking (progressive)
  - What did you used to drink in the past? And what do you drink now?

Edwards and Gross criteria for dependence syndrome

- Compulsion
  - Do you sometimes crave a drink?
  - Do you have a compulsive urge to drink?
- Tolerance
  - Does a drink have less of an effect on you than before?
  - Nowadays, do you need more alcohol to get drunk than you needed before?
- Withdrawal symptoms
  - What happens if you go without a drink for a day or two?
  - Have you ever had 'the shakes'?
  - If you don't drink for a day or two, do you experience any withdrawal symptoms such as sweating, shaking, weakness, headaches, feeling sick or pounding in your heart?
- Relief drinking
  - Do you need a drink first thing in the morning to steady your nerves?
  - Do you have to gulp the first few drinks of the day?
- Stereotyped pattern
  - Do you always drink in the same pub?
  - Do you always drink with the same company?
- Treatment and rapid reinstatement
  - Ask about details of treatment and details of any period of abstinence or binge drinking

- What helped you keep off drink?
- Have you ever had an extended period of time when you didn't drink?
- What happened to make you start drinking again?
- Have you ever gone to anyone for help with your drink problem?
- Have you ever been in hospital because of your drinking?
- Have you followed any detoxification programme?
  a. Was it completed or not?
  b. If not, what are the reasons?
- Primacy
  - How important is drink compared with other activities?
  - How often do you miss family and social commitments because of drinking?
  - Have you been giving primary importance to alcohol, and have you been neglecting other alternative pleasures or interests?

It is important to rule out mood and psychotic symptoms and also to rule out illicit drug abuse.

Assessing complications of alcohol misuse and assessing motivation

Physical health problems

- What do you think are the consequences of your drinking? (open question)
- Have you ever had any health problems due to drinking?
- Ask specific questions about:
  - Accidents and head injury
  - Memory problems
  - Blackouts, falls, fits
  - Loss of appetite, weight loss.

Mental health problems

- Have you ever had severe shaking, heard voices and seen things that were not there after heavy drinking?
- Also ask specifically about:
  - Anxiety, depression
  - Suicidal ideation/behaviour.

Social problems

Relationship difficulties with the partner, children, family members and friends:

- Has your drinking ever led to problems with your family, friends, work or the police?
- How has it affected your family life?
- Have you had any row or arguments with friends or mates?

Problems at the workplace:

- Has your drinking had an effect on your job like missing work, being late, Monday absences etc.

Financial problems:

- Have you ever had any financial problems because of your habit?

Legal problems – drink driving, drunk and disorderly behaviour, fights while drunk:

- Have you actually had an accident or hurt yourself?
- Have you ever been convicted of drink driving?
- Have you ever been arrested because of your drinking?

Insight and motivation

- Do you think that the problems you experience currently are related in any way to your drinking?
- What makes you feel that way and could you please explain that?
- Do you feel you have a problem with alcohol?
- What would you like to do?
- Have you ever thought of giving it up completely?
- What do you think will happen if you give up completely?

Eliciting illicit drug history

Open questions

- Are there any tablets or medicines that you take apart from those you get from your doctor?
- Is there anything that you buy from the chemist or get from friends?
- Have you ever used any recreational drugs or illegal drugs such as cannabis, cocaine/crack, amphetamines, speed, ecstasy, LSD or acid? (Ask about individual drugs by naming them.)
- What about tablets to 'settle your nerves' or to help you sleep?

Current usage

- What drugs are you using now?
- What is the frequency of use?

- What is the pattern of typical drug using?
- What is the amount of drug taken? (in appropriate measures)
- What effect are you seeking when using the drug?
- How much money do you spend in a day/week to get these drugs?
- What is the route of use – oral, smoked, snorted, injected? If injected, the following questions are useful to ask:
  - Are needles used?
  - Where are they obtained?
  - Are needles shared?
  - What sites are used for injection?
- What risky behaviour does the patient engage in?
  - Injecting and sharing needles?
  - Unsafe sex?
  - Sex for drugs?
- Is more than one drug used at a time?
- How is he/she financing the drug use?

Longitudinal history

Ask about the patient's age at first use of drugs, and when the patient started to use the drug regularly.

- When did it start?
- What was the first drug taken?
- Was it by your own free will or peer pressure?
- How did you progress to the current level?

Features of 'dependence syndrome'

- Compulsion
  - Do you sometimes crave drugs?
  - Do you have a compulsive urge to take drugs?
- Tolerance
  - Do you have to increase the amount of drugs that you take to get the same effect?
  - Does the same amount give you less of an effect than it used to?
- Withdrawal symptoms
  - If you don't take drugs for a day or two, do you experience any withdrawal symptoms? For example, if the patient takes heroin, ask about symptoms such as sweating, gooseflesh, running nose, watery eyes, etc.
  - Ask the patient to describe any withdrawal symptoms in their own words.

- Complications
  - Have you experienced any complications? Ask about physical, mental and social complications?
  - Have you ever worried about:
    a. Hepatitis B or C and HIV?
    b. Complications of injecting like infections, abscesses, septicaemia?
    c. Accidents, head injury, falls, fits?
    d. Anxiety, depression, hearing voices, seeing things?
    e. Financial problems?
    f. Arguments with friends or family members or work colleagues?
- Treatment
  - What is the patient's past experience of treatment for a drug problem?
  - Have you ever gone to anyone for help to come out of this?
  - Have you ever been in hospital for a drug problem?
  - Have there been any periods of abstinence when you were not using any drugs and if so, what has helped you achieve this?
  - What triggers have brought on this habit again?

Eliciting history of anxiety symptoms, panic attacks and phobias

- Have there been times when you have been very anxious or frightened? What was this like?
- Have you had the feeling that something terrible might happen?
- Have you had the feeling that you are always on the edge?
- Do you worry a lot about simple things?
- Tell me what made you feel so anxious? And tell me about your anxiety symptoms?
- How long have you been feeling so anxious?
- How does it interfere with your life and activities?
- Tell me about your sleep please. (Explore for sleep disturbance.)
- How has your sleep been recently?
- Have you had any trouble getting off to sleep?
- Are you sometimes afraid to go to sleep because you know that you will get unpleasant dreams?
- How has your concentration been recently?
- Do you lose your temper more often than you used to? (Irritability?)

Panic attacks

- Have you noticed any changes in your body when you feel anxious?

- Have you had times when you felt shaky, your heart pounded, you felt sweaty, dizzy and you simply had to do something about it?
- Were you getting butterflies in stomach, jelly legs, and trembling of hands?
- Have you ever had a panic attack? What was it like?
- What was happening at the time? Could you please describe it for me?
- How often do you get these attacks?
- How does it interfere with your life and activities?

Agoraphobia

- Do you tend to get anxious in certain situations such as travelling away from home or being alone?
- What about meeting people like in a crowded room?
- What about situations like being in a lift or tube?
- Do you tend to avoid any of these situations because you know that you'll get anxious?
- How much does it affect your life?

Social phobias

- Do any particular situations make you more anxious than others?
- Do you tend to get anxious when meeting people, e.g., going into a crowded room and making conversation?
- What about speaking to an audience? What about eating or drinking in front of other people?

Special phobias

- Do you have any special fears like people who are scared of cats or spiders or birds?

Avoidance

- Do you tend to avoid any of these situations because you know that you'll get anxious?
- Do you make any effort to avoid activities, places or people because you know that you will feel more anxious and embarrassed?
- What would you do? How does that make you feel?

Duration, effects and coping

- How long have you been feeling this way?
- What do you think might have caused this?

- How is it affecting your life?
- How do you manage to cope?
- Do you get any help?

Rule out co-morbidity:

- Depression
- Obsessional symptoms
- Anxious personality – would you say you were an anxious person?

Eliciting details of obsessive–compulsive symptoms

Obsessional thoughts

- Do any unpleasant thoughts/ideas keep coming back to your mind, even though you try hard not to have them?

OR

- Do you have any recurring thoughts, ideas, or images that you cannot get out of your mind?
- How often do you have these thoughts?
- Are these thoughts your own or are they put into your mind by some external force?
- Where do they come from?
- What is it like? How do you explain it?
- What do you do when you get these thoughts?
- Are they distressing and if so in what way?
- Is there anything you try to do to stop these thoughts?
- What happens when you try to stop them?

Compulsive acts

- Do you ever find yourself spending a lot of time doing the same thing over and over again even though you have already done it well enough? For example:
  - Do you spend a lot of time on personal cleanliness, like washing over and over even though you know that you're clean?
  - Does contamination with germs worry you?
  - Do you find that you have to keep on checking things that you know that you have already done? Like gas taps, doors, and switches?
- What happens when you try to stop doing this?
- Do you have to touch (or) count things many times?

- Do you have any other rituals?
- Do you find it difficult to make decisions even for simple trivial things? (Obsessional ruminations.)
- Do you have any impulses to do unwise things?
- What kind, and do you ever give in to these impulses?

Explore in detail about the symptom history, mode of onset, duration, precipitating factors and associated problems.

Duration, effects and coping

- How long have you been feeling this way?
- What do you think might have caused this?
- How is it affecting your life?
- How do you manage to cope?
- Do you get any help?

Co-morbidity

Ask about associated symptoms, such as:

- Depression, generalized anxiety, phobias.
- Anancastic personality traits – Do you tend to do things/keep things in an organized way?

Eliciting post-traumatic stress disorder history

Traumatic incident

Explore the details of the incident, in particular the perceived severity, and establish the level of distress and fear at the time of the event. Here, approach the patient empathetically as it is difficult to talk about traumatic incidents, and acknowledge the patient's distress.

- Could you describe the accident please?
- Find out about when it happened, how terrifying it was.
- Ask about any injuries, in particular head injury, loss of consciousness, whether any other person was injured, etc.
- Enquire about any blame, litigation, court cases and their outcome.

Core features

Core features of post-traumatic stress disorder are intrusions, avoidance, hyperarousal and emotional detachment and numbness.

Intrusions

- How often do you think about the accident?
- Do you sometimes feel as if the accident is happening again?
- Do you get flashbacks?
- Have you revisited the scene?
- Do you get any distressing dreams/nightmares of the event?
- What happens if you hear about an accident?

Avoidance

- How hard is it for you to talk about the accident?
- Have you been to the place where the accident happened?
- Do you deliberately try to avoid thinking about accidents?
- Do you make any effort to avoid the thoughts or conversations associated with the trauma? How would you do that?
- Do you make any effort to avoid activities, places or people that arouse recollection of the trauma?

Hyperarousal

- Have you had the feeling that you are always on the edge?
- Do you tend to worry a lot about things going wrong? (Feeling anxious?)
- Do you startle easily? (Enhanced startle response?)
- Tell me about your sleep please (explore for sleep disturbance).
- Are you sometimes afraid to go to sleep?
- How has your concentration been recently?
- How has your memory been lately?
- Tell me about your temper please (irritability).

Emotional detachment and numbness

- How do you feel in yourself generally?
- Have there been any changes in your feelings generally? (Emotional detachment?)
- How do you see the future?

Other issues

- Assess the mode of onset of symptoms, duration, progress, severity and frequency of current symptoms
- Distress and impairment of social functioning
  - I would like to know how your problems have been affecting you, your family and your social life
- Explore co-morbidity
  - Mood symptoms, especially depression and anxiety symptoms
  - Current coping mechanisms, including drugs and alcohol.

Eliciting eating disorder history

Psychological issues

- Do you think you have a problem with your weight and eating?
- How do you feel about your weight right now?
- What is your ideal weight?
- Why is this weight ideal for you?
- Are you satisfied with how you look?
- Do you feel fat? Do you feel ugly?
- How do you feel when you see your image in a mirror?
- Do you feel that you have a distorted body image? If so, in what way?
- Do you fear loss of control? What do you mean by that?
- What do you feel would happen if you did not control your weight or eating?

Eating issues

- What is a typical day's eating?
- Is there a pattern? Does it vary?
- Do you avoid any particular foods? And if so, why?
- Do you restrict fluids?

Binge eating

- Do you ever have times where you feel that your eating is out of control or seems excessive?
- Do you ever binge eat? (i.e., eat, during a short space of time, quantities of food that are definitely larger than most people would eat during a similar time and in similar circumstances)
- When did you first start binge eating?
- How often do you do it and why do you binge eat?
- Tell me about a typical binge? (obtain information about type of foods eaten, quantity of food, duration of the binge, vomiting or purging after the binge)
- How do you feel just before you binge?
- Can you identify any particular cause (e.g., feelings, stressors, social situations) that may trigger the binge?
- How do you feel while you are binge eating?
- How do you feel after bingeing?

Vomiting

- Have you ever had to make yourself sick? If so how?

- How often do you do this?
- Can you tell me why you make yourself vomit?

Laxatives, diuretics, emetics, appetite suppressants, exercise

- Often, many people with these problems use other methods to control their weight such as (give examples and ask specifically) taking laxatives, water pills, emetics and appetite suppressants.
- For what reason do you use it?
- Do you fast for a day or more?
- Do you exercise?
- How often do you exercise?
- Is this to burn off calories?
- Do you use exercise as a means of controlling your weight?

Physical symptoms

- Menstrual changes
  - When was your last period?
  - Are you menstruating regularly?
- Changes in libido
- Symptoms of anaemia: weakness, lethargy, constipation
  - Do you feel the cold badly?
  - Have you noticed any weakness in your muscles?
  - Have you fainted or had dizzy spells?
  - Have you noticed any palpitations?

Other issues

Explore:

- Any difficult situation at home or at work
- Current relationship
- Social activities and life in general
- Recent stressors.

Assessing insight

- You have described several symptoms namely... (repeat the symptoms) and what is your explanation of these experiences? Do you think that the symptoms were part of your nervous condition?
- Do you consider that you are ill in any way?

OR

- Do you think there is anything the matter with you?
- What do you think it is? Do you have a physical or mental illness?
- Could it be a nervous condition? What is it?
- Do you feel that you need help to deal with this problem?
- What kind of help do you think would be useful?
- Do you need treatment for a mental problem now?
- Why do you think that you have come into the hospital?
- What do you feel about being in hospital?
- Do you think that it has helped you to be here? If so, in what way?
- Has the medication been helpful?
- Do you think that medication helps you to remain well?
- Will you take the recommended medication for the future?
- Have any other treatments been helpful?

Eliciting history of premorbid personality

Open question

Start with open questions:

- How would you describe yourself as a person before you were ill?
- How do you think other people would describe you as a person?

Closed questions

Then ask closed questions about individual personality traits.

Cluster A (paranoid, schizoid, schizotypal)

- How do you get on with people? (paranoid)
- Do you trust other people? (paranoid)
- Would you describe yourself as a 'loner'? (schizoid)
- Have you always been able to make friends?
- Do you have any close friends? (schizoid)
- Do you indulge in fantasies? Sexual and non-sexual fantasies, daydreaming?

- Do you like to be around other people or do you prefer your own company?

Cluster B (antisocial, borderline and histrionic)

- What's your temper like? (antisocial, emotionally unstable)
- How do you deal with criticisms?
- Are you an impulsive person? (impulsive)
- Do you take responsibility for your actions? (antisocial, impulsive)
- Are you over-emotional (histrionic)?
- How do you cope with life? (borderline)
- How do you react to stress? (borderline)
- Do you maintain long-term relationships with people? (antisocial, borderline)
- Do you often feel that you are empty inside?

Cluster C (anxious, dependent and anancastic)

- Are you anxious or shy? (anxious/avoidant)
- Are you a worrier? (anxious, dependent)
- How much do you depend on others? (dependent)
- Would you describe yourself as a perfectionist? (anancastic)
- Do you tend to keep things in an orderly way? (anancastic)
- Do you have unusually high standards at work/home (anancastic)

Other questions

Enquire about:

- Predominant mood
  - Optimistic/pessimistic
  - Stable/prone to anxiety
  - Cheerful/despondent
- Interpersonal relationships
  - Current friendships and relationships
  - Previous relationship – ability to establish and maintain
  - Sociability – family, friends, work mates and superiors
- Coping strategies
  - How do you cope with problems?
  - When you find yourself in difficult situations, what do you do to cope?
- Personal interests – hobbies, leisure time
  - What sort of things do you like to do to relax?
- Beliefs – religious beliefs. Are you religious?
- Habits – food fads, alcohol, current/previous use of drugs, etc.

Dementia – history taking (collateral information)

The format given below can be used to elicit history and collateral information for all types of dementia and can be used in a wide variety of settings such as outpatient clinic, memory clinic, inpatient units and community assessments.

Introduce yourself to the patient's relative and address the main concerns:

- Please describe for me the problems your husband has been having? (Open question)
- Can you give me examples of his forgetfulness?
- Anything else you are concerned about?

Onset and progression:

- When did the symptoms start?
- What symptoms were noticed first?
- Did it start gradually or suddenly?
- Has it progressed gradually or suddenly?
- Are there any fluctuations?

Cognitive symptoms

Inquire about symptoms in all cognitive domains

Memory

(Make sure that you enquire about both short term and long term loss, if present)

Short-term memory:

- Can he remember things that happened in the last few minutes or in the day?
- Can you give me some examples?
  - Forgetting people's names?
  - Forgetting appointments or important dates?
  - Forgetting conversations he has had with people?
  - Forgetting where he has put things (misplacement of personal and household items)?
  - Repeating himself, asking the same question more than once?
  - Forgetting to take medication or taking it twice?

Long-term memory:

- Can he remember events that happened a few years ago?
- Can you please give me some examples?

- Does prompting or recognition help?
- Is it consistent or patchy?

Temporal and spatial disorientation

- Does he know the time of the day, the day of the week, date of the month, etc?
- How often does he lose his way at home or in the neighbourhood?
- What about getting lost on what are familiar routes?

Language difficulties

- How about the way he speaks?
- Does he have any word-finding problems?
- Can he understand when someone speaks to him?

Dyspraxia

- The memory problems that you describe, do they affect his ability to look after himself, or to do the things he used to?
- Does he have difficulty doing things for himself like maintaining personal hygiene, washing, cooking, laundry, etc? (Activities of daily living.)
- Does he have difficulty in cooking a meal or organizing payment of bills?
- Is he able to handle money?
- Can he do his own shopping?

Dyslexia, dysgraphia

- What about reading and writing?

Visuospatial difficulties, agnosia

- Does he have difficulty recognizing things, places or people?
- Does he have difficulty in recognizing familiar faces?

Judgement, decision making

- What about planning, making decisions, etc?
- Has he got difficulty in solving everyday problems that he used to solve?

Behavioural symptoms

- Has there been any change in his behaviour, such as being more irritable than usual?
- Have you noticed any change in personality that seems to have occurred recently?

- Ask about becoming aggressive frequently, episodes of violence and anger outbursts
- Also enquire about behaving inappropriately, social withdrawal, wandering at night time, disinhibited behaviour, repetitive behaviours, etc.

Psychological symptoms

- Inquire about symptoms of depression (low mood, crying spells) and anxiety.
- Also enquire about paranoia, auditory and visual hallucinations and other psychotic symptoms.

Physical symptoms

Ask briefly about:

- Sensory impairment
- Weakness of limbs
- Gait disturbance
- Parkinson's disease – any abnormal movements
- Incontinence.

Biological symptoms

Inquire about:

- Sleep disturbance and symptoms getting worse at night
- Appetite disturbance
- Loss of weight.

Risk assessment

- Fire risk – safety in the home, can use cooker safely, smoking, etc.
- Management of finances
- Inappropriate use of medication
- Risk of driving.

Other relevant factors in the patient's history

- Current medication
- Past medical history
  - High blood pressure
  - Diabetes
  - Thyroid disorders

- Infections
- Stroke
- Past psychiatric history: particularly depression
- Family history of dementia
- Risk factors for dementia
  - Alcohol
  - Head injury
- Personal history
  - Education
  - Occupation
  - Living situation.

Mini mental state examination

The areas to be covered are: Temporal orientation, spatial orientation, registration, attention, concentration, recall, naming, repetition, comprehension, reading, writing, copying.

Orientation to time

- What is the year? (1 score)
- What is the season? (1 score)
- What is the month? (1 score)
- What is the day of the week? (1 score)
- What is the date? (1 score)

Orientation to place

- What is the country? (1 score)
- What is the county/state/province? (1 score)
- What city are we in? (1 score)
- What is the name of the hospital or building? (1 score)
- What floor are we on? (1 score)

Registration

- Repeat till you remember: apple, table, penny. (3 score)

(The first repetition determines his/her score but keep saying them until he/she can repeat all 3, up to 6 trials.)

Attention and concentration

- Spell the word 'WORLD'; now try to spell it backwards D-L-R-O-W. (5 score)

Recall

- What were the three words that you were asked to remember? (3 score)

Comprehension

- Take this paper in your right hand, fold it in half and put it on the floor. (3 score)

Naming

- What is this called? (show a watch)
- What is this called? (show a pencil) (2 score)

Repetition

- Repeat after me 'No ifs, ands or buts'. (1 score)

Reading

- Read and do what is written down 'CLOSE YOUR EYES'. (1 score)

Writing

- Write a short sentence. (1 score)

Copying

Copy this drawing (2 interlocking pentagons). (1 score)

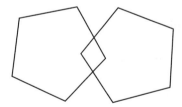

Detailed cognitive examination

A detailed cognitive assessment involves checking for:

- Orientation to time, place and person
- Attention
- Calculation
- Memory
- Language
- Visuospatial and visuoconstructive functions

- Executive functions
- Assessment of praxis.

Orientation to time, place and person

Orientation to time

- What is the year?
- What is the season?
- What is the month?
- What is the day of the week?
- What is the date?

Orientation to place

- What is the country?
- What is the county/state/province?
- What city are we in?
- What is the name of the hospital or building?
- What floor are we on?

Orientation to person

- Can you tell me your name (including surname)?
- How old are you?
- What is your occupation?

Attention and concentration

- Serial reversal tasks – spelling W-O-R-L-D backwards, serial 7s from 100; other tests include reciting months of the year backwards, days of the week backwards
- Calculations – ask the patient to perform mental arithmetic such as addition, subtraction, multiplication or division. For example, ask the patient to write down four or five numbers and add them up.

Memory

Working memory

- Forward digit span – a series of numbers is read to the subject who then repeats the numbers back. The numbers should be read evenly at one per second and start from three digits. The normal range is 6 ± 1.
- Backward digit span – the subject is asked to repeat the string of numbers backwards (e.g., the examiner reads 396 and the patient answers 693). The normal range is 5 ± 1.

Anterograde memory (new learning)

Registration and recall of three items:

- Ask if you can test the individual's memory. Name three objects (e.g., apple, table, penny) taking one second to say each one. Then ask the individual to repeat the names of all three objects.
- Ask for the three objects repeated above. What were the three objects I asked you to repeat a little while ago? Give 1 point for each correct object. (Recall should be tested five minutes after presenting the words.)

Registration and recall of a seven-item name and address:
'I am going to read you a name and address that I would like you to repeat after me. We will be doing it three times so that you have a chance to learn it and I will be asking you about it later.'
Then read out the following address:

John Brown
42, West Street, Luton
Bedfordshire

This can be recorded as a score out of 7 on the first learning trial, e.g., 4/7. Repeat the entire name and address in completion before the subject again tries to complete. Recall can be tested at 5–10 minutes. A score of 5 or less may give cause for concern if all seven items were learnt.

Retrograde memory (memory for personal events)

- Where did you grow up and go to school?
- When did you finish school?
- When did you get married?

Semantic memory (general events)

- Who is the current prime minister of the UK?
- Who is the previous prime minister of the UK?
- Who is the current president of the USA?
- Who is the previous president of the USA?
- What are the years of World War II?
- Has anything important happened in the world e.g. on September 11, 2001?
  - Description of any recent news events, e.g., political, sports events, accidents, catastrophes.

Language functions

Comprehension

- Simple commands, e.g., 'Close your eyes, touch your nose'.

Repetition

Sentences that are used for testing:

- Repeat 'No ifs, ands or buts'
- The orchestra played and the audience applauded.

Naming

- Point to two or three objects and ask patient to name them.
  - Ask the patient to name high frequency global names (such as, e.g., watch, jacket) and also more specific/lower frequency items (such as, e.g., label or winder) that are generally more difficult.

Word fluency

- Ask the patient to generate a list of as many animals as possible in one minute (normal: 15 in a category in one minute). Typical categories used to test include animals, fruits, vehicles.

Reading

- Show the individual the 'CLOSE YOUR EYES' message. Ask him or her to read the message.

Writing

- Ask the individual to write a sentence on a blank piece of paper. The sentence must contain a subject (real or implied) and a verb, and must be sensible.

Visuospatial and visuoconstructive functions

Tested by asking the subject to copy drawings or shapes which are three dimensional in nature (Figure 2).

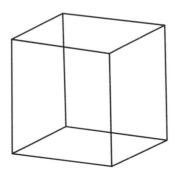

Clock drawing test

- Draw a circle and ask the subject to fill in numbers and hands to current time and tell the subject to set the time at 'ten' past 'eleven'.

In this task look for signs of neglect or of disorganization in the approach. This can indicate perceptual and perceptuomotor deficits, constructional apraxia and unilateral neglect.

Executive function

This involves frontal lobe functions that include verbal fluency, cognitive estimation, abstract thinking and reasoning, response inhibition, motor sequencing and programming (please read section 'Frontal lobe function testing' below).

Praxis

Ideomotor praxis

- Show me how you brush your teeth?
- Show me how you comb your hair?
- Show me how you cut paper with scissors?

Ideational praxis

- Ask the subject to perform a complex task with multiple steps, for example, placing a letter in an envelope, sealing it, addressing it, stamping it and then posting it.

Orobuccal praxis

Ask the subject to carry out specific movements on command, such as 'Stick out your tongue', 'Lick your lips', etc.

Frontal lobe function testing

Assessment of verbal fluency/category fluency

- The patient is asked to name as many words as possible beginning with either the letters 'F, A or S' in one minute. (Ideally all three ought to be tested.)

Normal subjects should produce at least 15 words for each letter. Less than 10 items is definitely abnormal.

Alternatively you can use a category (name as many animals as possible in one minute). Typical categories used to test include animals, fruits, vehicles etc.

Assessment of abstraction

- Proverb interpretation – ask the patient the meaning of two common proverbs:
  - Example 1: Too many cooks spoil the broth.
  - Example 2: A stitch in time saves nine.
- Similarities – the patient is asked to explain the similarities between things (use things that are routinely used):
  - Example 1: table and chair
  - Example 2: apple and orange
  - Example 3: glass and ice
- Cognitive estimation: ask the patient to make estimates such as:
  - What is the height of an average English man?
  - How many camels are there in England?

Coordinated movements (tests response inhibition and set shifting)

- Alternate sequence – an alternating sequence of squares and triangles is shown to the patient and they are asked to copy it (Figure 3).

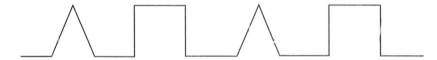

- Go/no-go test – ask the patient to place a hand on the table and to raise one finger in response to a single tap, while holding still in response to two taps. You tap on the under surface of the table to avoid giving visual cues.
- Luria three-step task – a sequence of hand positions is demonstrated which would be placing a fist, then edge of the palm and then a flat palm onto the palm of the opposite hand and repeating the sequence (fist-edge-palm). It can be demonstrated up to five times.

Frontal lobe release signs

- Glabellar tap – tap between the patient's eyebrows, which causes repeated blinking even after five or more taps, if it is positive.
- Primitive reflex – this would include the grasp reflex in which you stroke the patient's palm while distracting the patient and watch for involuntary grasping; and the pouting reflex in which you tap on a spatula on the patient's lips, resulting in pouting. Both reflexes can be subtle.

Suicide risk assessment

Perform suicide risk assessment in Miss X, a young woman admitted to the medical ward following an overdose.

Areas to be concentrated upon

1. Obtain more information about the overdose.
2. Evaluate the degree of suicidal intent and seriousness of the attempt.
3. Investigate symptoms of depression/psychosis or other forms of mental illness.
4. Assess current mental state including suicidal thoughts.
5. Obtain past history and background information.
6. Assess coping methods and ability to seek help.

Step 1: Obtain the following information about the overdose

- How many tablets were taken?
- What type of tablets was taken?
- When was the overdose taken?
- How was the medication obtained?
- Where was the patient when she took the overdose?
- How and by whom was she discovered?
- What did she do after the overdose?
- How did she end up coming to hospital?
- Did she take anything else with the tablets, for example, alcohol?
- *Why* did she take the overdose? (or)
  What was the event leading up to the suicidal act? (or)
  What made her think of harming herself? (or)
  What sorts of things have been worrying her?

If the patient is not forthcoming with all the details, use more closed questions and also examples, such as:

- Conflict in a close relationship
- A major loss or separation
- Family disharmony
- Difficulties at work
- Financial worries/housing
- Health problems
- Redundancy or legal problems
- Was there any direct gain (e.g., patient in custody at the time of the act)?

Step 2: Assessment of the degree of suicidal intent and seriousness of the attempt

A detailed assessment should include evaluation of the characteristics of the attempt.

Remember 4 Ps:

- Planning/impulsivity
- Performance in isolation or in front of others
- Preparations made prior to the act
- Precautions to avoid discovery of others.

The degree of suicidal intent

- Did the person plan the attempt carefully or was it impulsive?
- Did she take any steps towards doing this? (e.g., getting pills)
- Was anyone else actually present at the time?
- Did she convey her suicidal intent to others?
- Where did the act take place?
- Would she have anticipated being found?
- Did she take measures to avoid discovery?
- Did she make any preparations like arranging for the care of children etc?
- Did she leave any *suicide note*?

The seriousness of the attempt

- What method was used?
- Did the person understand the consequences of the method she used?
  - For example, was the person taking an overdose aware of the actions of the drug and did she believe that the dose taken would be fatal?
  - Did she take all the tablets or did she leave a few behind?
  - What are the problems experienced by the patient currently?

Step 3: Explore depressive symptoms and or psychotic symptoms with duration and their impact or current functioning

See *Eliciting symptoms of depression and suicidality* in Chapter 9.

Step 4: Assess current mental state: mocd and hopelessness

- How do you feel in yourself?
- How do you see the future?
- Do you still feel that life is not worth living?

Suicidal thoughts and plans

- Do you still have thoughts of harming yourself in any way?
- What do you think you might do?
- Have you made any plans?
- When are you intending to do it?
- What prevents you from doing it?

Step 5: Past history and background information

- Does she have a past history of suicidal behaviour?
- Does she suffer from a mental illness, for example, depression, psychosis, anxiety disorder, borderline personality disorder?
- Is there a history of non-compliance with treatment?
- Does she abuse alcohol or drugs?
- Is there a family history of mental illness, alcohol or substance abuse, violence or suicidal behaviour?

Step 6: Coping methods and ability to seek help

- What were her reactions to previous stresses, failures and losses?
- What does she usually do when there is a problem?
- How does she usually cope?
- With whom does she share her worries?
- How supportive are family and friends?
- Does she get any help?
- In the past, did anyone offer her any help? How did she find it?

Summary of assessment

By the end of the assessment, we should be able to answer the following questions, which might help in decision making and formulating a safe management plan:

- Is there evidence of mental illness?
- Is there ongoing suicidal intent?
- Are there non-mental health issues, which can be addressed?
- What is the level of social support available?

Suicide risk factors

Static and stable risk factors

- Age – older age
- Sex – male

- Marital status – divorced > single > widowed > married
- Childhood adversity
- Family history of suicide
- History of mental disorder
- Previous hospitalization
- History of substance use disorder
- Personality disorder/traits – impulsive or aggressive.

Dynamic risk factors

- Active psychological symptoms
- Active suicidal ideation, communication and intent
- Feelings of guilt, hopelessness, worthlessness and depressive features
- Treatment adherence
- Psychosocial stressors
- Alcohol and substance misuse
- Psychiatric admission and discharge
- Social support – housing, employment, financial status, family support.

Future risk factors for suicide

- Access to preferred methods of suicide
- Future stressors in life
- Future service contact
- Future response to drug treatment
- Future response to psychosocial intervention.

Deliberate self-harm

Risk factors

- Sex – female
- Age – younger age of onset
- Marital status – divorced > single > widowed > married
- Lower social class
- Unemployed
- Personality disorder
- Substance misuse.

Risk factors for repetition of self-harm

- Previous history of self-harm
- Alcohol and drug abuse
- Criminal record and history of violence

- Personality disorder – antisocial personality
- Psychiatric treatment
- Unemployment
- Lower social class
- High suicidal intent
- Hopelessness
- Non-compliance with treatment.

The association between suicide and mental illness is given in Table 9.1.

TABLE **9.1** Association between suicide and mental illness

Illness	Percentage of people with this illness who commit suicide	Percentage of people who commit suicide who have this illness
Schizophrenia	10	5
Depression	15	70
Alcoholism	15	15

Violence-risk assessment

Task: Mr. W is a 45-year-old gentleman who has a diagnosis of paranoid schizophrenia. He has past history of violence to others when unwell and he has recently assaulted a neighbour. His care-coordinator has arranged for an assessment with you to assess his current risk of harm to others.

Areas to be concentrated upon

1. Obtain previous history of violence, the severity of the violence and the context in which the violence occurred.
2. Assess current violent impulses and fixed thoughts to harm anybody.
3. Explore the current possibility of being acutely unwell mentally and being non-compliant with medication.
4. Enquire about current alcohol and drug use.

Step 1: Previous history of violence

- Can you describe the incident that happened recently when you lost your control and became violent?
- What caused the incident in the first instance? What are the triggers for the violent outburst?
- Is it associated with acts of violence to people, property or both?
- Was it just verbal aggression or did you physically hit somebody?
- Did the incident result in injury to others?

- Did you use any weapon during this incident?
- What were you feeling at the time of the violence?
- Is there remorse following the outburst?

Explore whether the patient has history of violence, such as hurting others, fights, trouble with the police, etc., and also enquire about family history of violence.

- Are you the sort of person who has trouble controlling your anger?
- Have you found yourself hitting people when you are angry?
- Have you found yourself damaging property when you are angry?
- What is the most violent thing that you have ever done?

Step 2: Current violent impulses

- Is there anything about the present situation that makes you feel like damaging things or hitting people now?
- Do you feel that you might damage things now?
- Do you feel that you might hit people now?
- Are you angry at anyone?
- Who are you angry at?
- Are you thinking about hurting the person mentioned?
- When do you think you might hurt them?
- Where will you do this?
- How long have you been thinking this way?
- How do you intend to harm them, and how serious might it be?
- Do you feel a strong urge to do so?
- Do you have access to weapons, etc?
- Are you able to control these thoughts about hurting this person?
- Do you think that you would be able to stop yourself from hurting the person if you wanted to?

Step 3: Look for psychotic symptoms and compliance to treatment plan

- Is there something or someone trying to control you?
- Do you feel under the control of some force or power other than yourself as though you are a robot or a zombie without a will of your own?
- Do you feel that forces beyond your control dominate your mind?
- Are thoughts put in your head that are not your own?
- Do you think that there might be people who intend to do you harm?
- Who are they? What do you intend to do about it?
- Enquire about command hallucinations and hallucinations of a derogatory or threatening content (see *Eliciting history of hallucinations* in Chapter 9).

- Explore delusions of persecution and reference (see *Eliciting details of delusions* in Chapter 9).
- Have you been taking your medication regularly?
- Do you think that you might be unwell at the moment?
- In what way do you think you are unwell?

Step 4: Substance use – enquire about current alcohol and drug use

- Have you used any alcohol over the past few days?
- Have you used other drugs over the past few days?
- Were you using drugs or alcohol in the past when you were violent?
- Have you taken anything now?

Potential risk factors for violence

- Being male
- Low intelligence
- Living or growing up in a violent subculture
- Past history of violence
- History of violence in the family
- History of poor impulse control
- Easy access to weapons and victims
- Abuse of drugs or alcohol.

untml:cut/>

10

Direct observation of procedural skills (DOPS)

Electroconvulsive therapy administration

Task: You are requested to administer electroconvulsive therapy (ECT) to Mr X, who has consented to the procedure.

Suggested approach

- Greet and introduce yourself.
- Obtain permission before you proceed.
- Check that it is the correct 'patient' and confirm the identity of the patient.
- Check documentation to see that the patient has consented and the *ECT consent form* has been duly signed, or if on a section of the Mental Health Act, the appropriate forms have been filled in.
- Ask for consent again and briefly explain the procedure.
- Check that the pre-ECT form has been filled in, with emphasis on *nil by mouth* for at least 6 hours prior to ECT.
- Check that the *physical examination* has been done prior to ECT, all necessary *investigations* duly completed and anaesthetist's opinion obtained.
- Check the *medical notes* to ensure that the psychiatric team has seen the patient after the last treatment to record progress and any adverse effects of ECT (if any after the last treatment).
- Check the *treatment card* to check for current medications.
- Make sure that the *appropriate dose has been set up*. Once the patient is anaesthetized the ECT electrodes should be placed accordingly and the treatment administered.
- Indicate the electrode placement for unilateral and bilateral ECT (see below).
- During treatment, also observe the nature, type and duration of the seizures.

- Make sure that you have documented the current used, type and duration of seizures, any complications that arose, in the medical notes and on the ECT form.
- Make sure that the patient is taken to the recovery room accompanied by a nurse and the vital signs are being monitored.
- Comment on your findings to the examiner as well as giving the EEG interpretation.
- Thank the examiner at the end and leave the station.

Electrode positions

Bilateral: 4 cm above the midpoint of the line between external auditory meatus and the lateral angle of the eye.

Unilateral: The first electrode is placed on the non-dominant side, 4 cm above the midpoint of the line between external angle of the eye and the external auditory meatus. The second electrode is placed 10 cm above the first, vertically above the meatus on the same side.

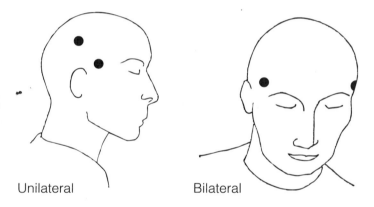

Unilateral   Bilateral

EEG interpretation

Look for the stimulus on the EEG record. The EEG usually develops patterned sequences consisting of high-voltage sharp waves and spikes, followed by rhythmic slow waves that end abruptly in a well-defined endpoint.

Key points about ECT treatment

Royal College recommendations

Bilateral ECT

- The optimal frequency is twice per week.
- The initial electrical dose should be at least 50% above the initial seizure threshold (i.e., one and a half times).

Unilateral ECT

- The optimal frequency is twice per week.
- The initial electrical dose should be at least three times above the initial seizure threshold.

ECT machine

- The treatment is administered using a constant-current brief pulse machine, which can offer a wide range of electrical dose from 25–50 millicoumbs to 750–800 millicoumbs.

Seizure duration

- ECT should induce the type of generalized cerebral seizure activity and the seizure activity could be questioned if the convulsion lasted less than 15 seconds or the EEG recording showed seizure activity lasting less than 25 seconds (Scott and Lock, 1995)

Seizure threshold

- This increases with age.
- It is higher in men than in women.
- It is increased by the use of anticonvulsants and benzodiazepines.
- It may increase during a course of ECT.

Contraindications to ECT

There are relatively few contraindications to ECT, including the following:

- Recent cerebrovascular accident (CVA; within 1 month)
- Recent myocardial infarction (within 3 months)
- Raised intracranial pressure
- Uncontrolled cardiac failure
- Untreated cerebral aneurysm
- Untreated phaeochromocytoma
- Acute respiratory infection
- Unstable major fracture.

Investigations to be completed prior to ECT

- Full blood count
- Urea and electrolytes
- Blood pressure and weight
- Urinalysis

- Blood sugar levels (if urinalysis is positive)
- ECG for patients with known cardiovascular disease, all patients over the age of 50 years and those with diabetes aged over 40 years.
- Chest X-ray for patients with suspected chest infection, congestive heart failure and cardiomegaly.

Checklist for all patients scheduled for ECT

- Identity (name band with hospital number)
- Inpatient/outpatient
- Legal status
- Consent
- Fasting state (patients should take no food for 6 hours and drink only moderate volumes of clear fluids until 2 hours before treatment)
- Details of any premedication.

Recovery area (Royal College ECT Guidelines)

It should be equipped with:

- Pulse oximetry
- Sphygmomanometer
- Suction with suitable cannulae/catheters
- Oxygen supply, tubing, mask or nasal cannulae.

Cardiopulmonary resuscitation (basic life support)

Task: Perform CPR on this collapsed patient on your ward.

OR

Please provide basic life support (BLS) to this patient who has been found collapsed in the ward.

Please follow these steps in strict order:

1. Is it safe to approach? Is there any trauma?
2. After assuming that there is no trauma and the patient is safe, go near the manikin. Shake him by his shoulders and ask loudly at the same time – 'Hello, hello, can you hear me?' or 'Are you OK?'
3. If no response, shout for help – 'Help, Help!' Often the dummies in this station are clad with jumpers or other clothes, so remember to undress the dummy above the waist.
4. Check for a patent airway to rule out any foreign body secretions (etc.). If the airways are clear, tilt the head and lift the chin.

5. Now bend down by the side of the mannequin's face and look, listen and feel for no more than 10 seconds. Look for chest movement, listen at the victim's mouth for breath sounds and feel the air on your cheek.
6. If there are no signs of breathing, activate the emergency alarm system and dial '999'.
7. Start chest compression as follows; kneel by the side of the victim, place the heel of one hand in the centre of the victim's chest, place the heel of your other hand on top of the first hand, interlock the fingers of your hands, position yourself vertically above the victim's chest and with your arms straight, press down on the sternum to a depth of 4–5 cms. After 30 compressions, open the airway again using head tilt and chin lift.
8. Now give two effective rescue breaths – maintain the head tilt, chin lift position and then pinch the nose and purse your lips tightly on the mannequin's lips. Blow as forcefully as possible, while keeping an eye on the chest expansion. If there is no chest expansion, then either your technique is wrong or the airway is not open.
9. Then return your hands without delay to the correct position on the sternum and give a further 30 chest compressions.
10. Continue with chest compressions and rescue breaths in a ratio of 30:2 for at least 2 minutes.
11. Stop to recheck the victim only if he starts breathing normally. Otherwise, do not interrupt resuscitation.
12. Repeat the same cycle (30 chest compressions: 2 rescue breaths) until:
    – Patient responds
    – Help arrives
    – Or you are exhausted.

Once the patient is responsive, put him in the left lateral position, i.e., the *recovery position.*

A little modification is needed for some special situations such as:

● In cases of trauma, we do not tilt the head in case the cervical spine is injured. Instead we give a jaw thrust to open the airway.

Extrapyramidal side effects – physical examination

This would include:

● Akathisia (motor restlessness)
● Dystonia (uncontrolled muscular contraction)
● Pseudoparkinsonian features – tremor, rigidity, bradykinesia, mask-like facies and festinate gait
● Tardive dyskinesia (abnormal movements).

Suggested approach

- Greet the patient and introduce yourself.
- Address the patient's concerns first.
- Ask the patient briefly about any abnormal movements like slowness, stiffness, shakiness, feeling of inner restlessness and any other body movements that bother the patient.
- Explain briefly what you are going to do, and ask for consent. (Obtain permission before you proceed.)
- Ensure that the patient knows that during this examination you will be testing his hands, legs, and mouth and that you will make him walk to observe his gait.
- Observe the patient at rest for a few seconds.
- Ask the patient whether there is anything in his or her mouth and, if so, to remove it.
- Ask if he or she wears dentures. Ask whether teeth or dentures bother the patient now.
- Ask whether the patient notices any movements in his or her mouth, face, hands or feet. If yes, ask the patient to describe them and to indicate to what extent they are bothered by them.
- Ask the patient to open his or her mouth. (Observe the tongue at rest within the mouth.) Do this twice.
- Ask the patient to protrude his or her tongue. (Observe abnormalities of tongue movement.) Do this twice.
- Have the patient sit in chair with hands on knees, legs slightly apart and feet flat on floor. (Look at the entire body for movements while the patient is in this position. Observe for 15 seconds.)
- Ask the patient to sit with hands hanging unsupported – if male, between his legs, if female and wearing a dress, hanging over her knees. (Observe hands and other body areas for at least 15 seconds.)
- Ask the patient to tap his or her thumb with each finger as rapidly as possible for 10–15 seconds, first with the right hand, then with the left hand. (Observe facial, hand and leg movements.)
- Flex and extend the patient's left and right arms, one at a time.
- Ask the patient to stand up. (Observe the patient for 15 seconds. Observe all body areas again, hip included.)
- Ask the patient to extend both arms out in front, palms down. (Observe trunk, legs and mouth.)
- Have the patient walk a few paces, turn, and walk back to the chair. (Observe hands and gait.) Do this twice.

11

Sub-specialities

Child psychiatry

Interviewing the family

It is advisable to see the child or adolescent with all members of the family.

Enquire about the presenting problem and try to obtain a *full description* of the problem behaviour from parents, teachers, child, etc. It should include:

- The mode of onset or evolution of the presenting problem
- The nature and severity of the presenting problem
- Frequency
- The setting in which the problem behaviour manifests, e.g., home environment or at school
- The effect of it on siblings, family members, friends, school, attitude of others to the child's behaviour and the way that the parents deal or react with the problem behaviour
- Also enquire about other current problems or complaints.

Then try to obtain more history and, in any child psychiatry case, remember to obtain the following information in the history:

- Birth history – prenatal, perinatal and postnatal history
- Developmental history milestones (cognitive, languages, motor and social skills)
- History of serious childhood illness/hospitalizations
- Childhood neurotic traits (temper tantrums, enuresis, thumb sucking, nail biting, etc.)
- Losses/separation
- Problems at home: abuse – physical emotional and sexual; other difficult situation at home including parental disharmony and sibling rivalry; quality of parental and parent–child relationship

- Problems at school – teasing, bullying, poor academic performances, change of school, extra help, learning support, etc.
- Problems with peers being bullied/exposed to antisocial behaviour, drugs, etc.
- Recent stressful events
- Rule out the possibility of secondary gain for the problem behaviour.

Developmental history and parental relationship issues may be best obtained from parents.

Interviewing the child

Young children should be invited to play using age-appropriate toys, which would help to establish rapport and gain the child's confidence.

It would be more appropriate to begin the interview well away from the presenting problems by enquiring about friends, siblings, school, interests, hobbies, etc.

Then it would be useful to enquire about the following:

- The child's view of the problem
- Mood – any particular worries and/or fears
- Sleep and appetite
- Relationships with siblings and family members
- Relationship with friends or peers at school
- Difficulties at school – bullying, etc
- Fantasy life
- Abnormal experiences
- Suicidality.

Mental state examination

- Observe the child's appearance, behaviour, nutritional state
- Activity level, fidgetiness, involuntary movements
- Look for evidence of neglect, bruising, etc
- Habits and mannerisms
- Rapport, eye contact and spontaneous talk
- Mood – observe for signs of sadness, misery, tension, and anxiety
- Look for the presence of delusion, hallucination, thought disorder
- Level of awareness and evidence of absence seizures or minor epilepsy
- Also look for *the child's relationship with parents*, *interactions*, resentment and ease of separation; if siblings can be present, then their behaviour and interaction can also be evaluated
- It is also important to observe the pattern of interaction and emotional atmosphere of family, and also observe the ease of communication between family members.

Other assessments

Physical examination – usually have a parent present.

Psychological assessment – measures of intelligence and educational achievements are often valuable.

Key points

Depression

- Psychological treatments should always be considered as first line treatment for children with depressive illness.
- If pharmacological treatment is necessary, then fluoxetine hydrochloride (10–20 mg/day) is the treatment of choice.
- If there is no adequate response to fluoxetine hydrochloride and drug treatment is still considered to be necessary, then alternative SSRIs such as citalopram or sertraline hydrochloride should be tried cautiously.
- Paroxetine hydrochloride is specifically contraindicated due to increased risk of suicide.
- Severe depression that is unresponsive to other treatments, or life threatening, may respond to ECT. It should not be used in children under the age of 12 years.
- Early treatment with mood stabilizers should be considered, as up to a third of patients who have suffered an episode of depression will have a diagnosis of bipolar disorder within 5 years.

Anxiety disorders

- Psychological treatments such as CBT should always be considered as first line treatment for children with anxiety disorders.
- If pharmacological treatment is necessary, then SSRIs are first line agents.

Psychotic disorder

- Schizophrenia is rare in children but the incidence increases rapidly in adolescence.
- The treatment algorithms for treating psychosis in children and adolescents are the same as those for adult patients.
- However, weight gain may be more pronounced in children than in adults.
- First line – atypical antipsychotics:
  - Risperidone 2–4 mg/day
  - Olanzapine 2.5–15 mg/day
  - Quetiapine fumarate 100–400 mg/day
  - Amisulpride 100–400 mg/day.

Bipolar illness

- Valproate is usually the medication of first choice, followed by lithium and then carbamazepine:
  - Sodium valproate 500–2000 mg/day
  - Carbamazepine 100–600 mg/day.
- Valproate is effective in approximately 50% of acute manic or mixed episodes.
- Open label study supports the efficacy of olanzapine in acute mania.
- Adolescents often respond poorly to monotherapy and may need combination treatment.
- Lamotrigine could be used in treatment resistant depressive episodes.

Obsessive–compulsive disorder

- The treatment of OCD in children follows the same principle as in adults.
- Sertraline hydrochloride from 6 years and fluvoxamine malate from 8 years are the only SSRIs licensed in UK for the treatment of OCD in children.

Attention deficit hyperactivity disorder

- According to NICE guidance, methylphenidate hydrochloride is recommended for use as part of a comprehensive treatment programme for children with a diagnosis of attention deficit hyperactivity disorder (ADHD). The diagnosis should be based on a timely comprehensive assessment conducted by a child- and adolescent-psychiatrist or paediatrician with expertise in ADHD.
- Drug treatment should only be part of the treatment plan, and appropriate psychological, psychosocial and behavioural interventions should be put in place.
- Methylphenidate hydrochloride should be used as first line treatment. Start with 5–10 mg in the morning, and 5–10 mg at mid-day can be added; a late dose should be avoided as it can cause insomnia. The dosage can be titrated up to a maximum of 60 mg/day in divided doses using weekly increments of 5–10 mg.
- Side effects – loss of appetite and weight loss, nausea, vomiting, insomnia, anxiety, dysphoria, headaches, raised blood pressure and, rarely, tics.
- Growth retardation may be a long-term side effect of high doses over longer periods.
- Recommended monitoring – blood pressure, pulse, height and weight; monitor for insomnia, mood and appetite changes and the development of tics regularly.

- Monitor response using Connor's rating scale.
- Discontinue if no benefits are seen in 1 month.
- Methylphenidate hydrochloride sustained release tablets – start initially on 18 mg in the morning, titrated up to a maximum of 54 mg.
- Methylphenidate hydrochloride is not currently licensed for children under the age of 6 years.
- Other drugs that could be used would include dexamphetamine sulfate and atomoxetine.
- Atomoxetine should be started at 40 mg, which should be increased to 80 mg after 1 week. The once daily dosing is convenient for use in school children.
- Monitoring of liver function tests (LFTs) is advisable for children on atomoxetine.

Autistic spectrum disorder

- SSRIs may be effective in ameliorating repetitive and aggressive behaviour (open case series).
- Risperidone has been shown to be probably effective in the treatment of hyperactivity, repetitive behaviour and aggression in children with autistic spectrum disorder (Barnard et al. 2002).

Tourette's syndrome

- Risperidone and sulpiride have been shown to be effective and well tolerated.
- Other drugs that could be used are clonidine hydrochloride, haloperidol and pimozide.

Aggression/acute behavioural disturbance

- Low dose risperidone (0.25–2mg/day) or haloperidol could be tried.
- However, haloperidol tends to be poorly tolerated by children and risperidone can cause significant extrapyramidal side effects (EPSEs) in young people.
- Other atypicals could be tried but can cause considerable weight gain.

Common psychological intervention used in child psychiatry

Behavioural therapy

Behavioural methods are used to encourage new behaviour by positive reinforcement (e.g., praise, rewards) and modelling, and efforts are made to remove any factors in the child's environment that are reinforcing unwanted behaviour through negative reinforcement (e.g., by removing the child's privileges).

Functional behaviour analysis is performed to analyse the *ABC* (antecedents, behaviour and consequences) with the help of parents. Parents are taught how the child's unacceptable behaviour may be reinforced unintentionally by paying attention to it, and they are also taught how to reinforce normal behaviour by praise or rewards and how to eliminate unwanted behaviour by removing the child's privileges.

Cognitive therapy

It is useful mainly for older and school-age children who have the capabilities to describe their problems and who can learn to control their ways of thinking that give rise to symptoms and problem behaviour; the methods generally resemble those used with adults. The most common targets of CBT and social skills therapies for children are aggressive behaviour, emotional dysregulation, problem solving, social interactions and self evaluation.

Family therapy

'Symptoms' of the child are often considered as an 'expression' of malfunctioning of the family, which is the primary focus of treatment. Therefore, both parents are involved often together with the child and may be joined by other children and members of the extended family. The goals to be obtained would include:

- Improved communication within the family
- Improved autonomy for each member
- Improved agreement about roles and reduced conflict.

Parent management training

The aim is to improve the skills of parents with deficient parenting skills and is mainly used to assist parents of children with behavioural problems that require special parenting skills, for example, the parents of children with conduct disorder or hyperactivity.

These programmes use the behavioural principles as explained above. The parents are provided with written information and videotapes showing other parents applying these behavioural principles. It also involves teaching good parenting skills that include:

- Promoting a positive relationship with the child
- Using praise and rewards to increase desirable sociable behaviour
- Setting clear rules and directions

- Using consistent and calmly executed consequences for unwanted behaviour
- Reorganizing the child's play to prevent problems.

Teacher training and interventions in school

Teachers are taught techniques for use with children in their class and focus on interventions to promote positive behaviour.

The important targets of classroom techniques would be:

- Promoting positive behaviour and following established class rules and procedures
- Preventing problem behaviour and preventing the escalation of angry behaviour and acting out
- Teaching social and emotional skills such as problem solving and conflict resolution.

Multi-systemic therapy

- The intervention model with the most empirical support for treating children and adolescents with conduct disorder is multisystemic therapy (MST).
- Problem behaviours are *conceptualized* as being linked with individual characteristics and with various aspects of the multiple systems in which the child is embedded, including the family, peers, schools and neighbourhood.
- On a highly individualized basis, treatment goals are developed in collaboration with the *family*, and systemic *strengths* (e.g., an aptitude for sports or music) are used as levers for therapeutic change.
- Specific interventions used in MST are based on the best of the empirically validated treatment approaches, such as CBT and the pragmatic family therapies. Specific interventions are designed to promote responsible behaviour and reduce irresponsible behaviour.
- Intervention requires daily or weekly effort by parents and is designed to promote and empower parents and families to address their children's needs across multiple contexts and resolve future difficulties.
- The therapy is given for 3 months and then stopped.
- The progress is monitored on a weekly basis, which enables barriers to improvement to be addressed immediately. The parents and teenagers fill in weekly questionnaires on whether they have been receiving therapy as planned.
- The primary goals of MST are to reduce rates of antisocial behaviour in the adolescent and reduce out-of-home placements.

Social interventions

Remember 5 Ss:

- Special education and teaching to remedy backwardness in reading, writing and arithmetic skills
- Social worker – family assessment, individual counselling for the child and members of the family, arrangements for special care, finances and accommodation
- Support – increased support to parents and teachers
- Social activities – more indoor and outdoor activities at school and joining social clubs
- Substitute care – respite care, residential care, fostering, day-patient and inpatient care.

Learning disability

The assessment of the learning-disabled person involves six different steps:

- Obtaining history
- Physical examination
- Mental state examination
- Developmental assessment
- Functional behavioural assessment
- Interaction between the learning-disabled person and the family and the social support systems and other aspects of adjustment.

History

When obtaining history, it is important to pay attention to the following areas:

- Is there any family history suggesting an inherited disorder?
- Enquire about abnormalities in the pregnancy.
- Enquire about difficulties during the delivery of the child.
- Ascertain the dates of passing developmental milestones.
- Enquire about associated medical conditions such as epilepsy, cerebral palsy, etc.

Therefore developmental and personal history should include:

- Antenatal complications, maternal illness, exposure to medication and toxins, drug and alcohol misuse
- Perinatal history – mode of delivery, duration of labour, complications during labour, was resuscitation needed, birth weight, examination of birth records (weight, head circumference, length and Apgar score)
- Immediate postnatal period – infections, hospitalizations
- Childhood history – weight gain, growth pattern, feeding and sleeping patterns; early milestones – cognitive, language, motor and social skills; history of childhood illnesses and accidents
- Past medical history, including epilepsy, medications, infections, surgery
- Family history – parents' ages, consanguinity, family history of learning disabilities (LDs), specific cognitive impairments, congenital abnormalities, medical, neurological or psychiatric disorders.

Physical examination

- Look for physical signs and for evidence of dysmorphic features suggesting one of the many specific syndromes such as Down's syndrome, fragile X syndrome, etc.

- Perform a full physical examination including detailed neurological examination for localizing signs.
- Look for impairments of vision and hearing and if suggested by the history and examination, then ophthalmological and audiological examinations should be arranged.
- Look for features of self-injury.
- Look for the presence of tics, rituals and obsessions.
- Look for the presence of seizure-like movements and stereotypic behaviours.

Mental state examination

In those who are able to communicate well, the MSE does not differ significantly from individuals without LD. However, in those with limited or no verbal skills, detailed observation may be necessary. Serial assessments may be required to gather all the information due to poor attention and concentration.

Behavioural observations by family members and carers are often most helpful.

Developmental assessment

This is based on a combination of clinical experience and standardized methods of measuring cognitive, language, motor and social skills. Some commonly used instruments would include Vineland social maturity scale, the British ability scales and differential ability scales, the adaptive behaviour scale and the Portage guide to early education.

Functional behavioural assessment

This is based on observations made by the family members and carers of the person's ability to care for himself, his communication abilities, ability to interact socially, sensory motor skills and relationships with others.
The person's level of functioning may be assessed using:

- IQ assessment
- Type of schooling
- Daily living skills.

Interactions

Finally, it important to analyse the *interaction* between the learning-disabled person and the family and the social support systems, as well as other aspects of *adjustment, such as* making relationships and learning new skills.

If the person has poor communication abilities, then most of the information is obtained from the informants such as parents, teachers and carers.

Investigations

- Standard routine tests would include FBC, U&Es, LFTs, TFTs, glucose, infection screening (blood and urine) and serology for TORCH infections (Toxoplasmosis, Rubella, Cytomegalovirus, Herpes simplex and HIV)
- X-rays and ultrasound (cardiac/abdominal) indicated, if dysmorphic features are present
- Arrange for screening tests of blood and urine if metabolic disorder is suspected
- Arrange for karyotyping if genetic disorder is suspected
- Other more detailed investigation such as CT, MRI, EEG and functional imaging to be considered, if history and examination warrants it.

Challenging behaviour

The assessment of challenging behaviour relies on information from the individual, family members, carers, teachers and other professionals involved in his/her care. In those individuals with limited or no verbal skills, behavioural observations and recent changes that have been experienced should be taken into consideration, and collateral information from regular carers plays a major role in the assessment and management of such individuals.

The assessment should focus on identifying the possible common causes of challenging behaviour.

Common causes of challenging behaviour

- Presence of psychiatric disorder – depression, psychosis, ADHD, etc.
- Presence of physical disorder – pain and discomfort, infections, constipation, epilepsy, cerebral palsy, etc.
- Side effects of medication, especially psychotropic medications
- Environmental factors – change in environment/carers
- Difficulties in communication (frustration)
- Sensory deficits, such as vision or hearing impairment
- Desire to escape unpleasant situations
- Psychosocial factors, such as bereavement/disrupted family, recent stressful events; adverse experiences such as social rejection, neglect, physical, emotional or sexual abuse
- Poor temperament, particularly high emotionality, poor sociability and high activity.

Assessment

- Identify the problem behaviour.
- Identify the possible precipitants and exacerbating factors.
- When was it first identified?
- What is the duration of the problem behaviour?
- In what situation does it occur and what form does it take?
- How is the problem managed?
- What are the alleviating factors?
- Explore the possibility of recent environmental changes.
- Explore the possibility of recent physical changes.

Management

Following the assessment, the management plan should be tailored according to the needs of the individual patient, and specific factors should be addressed, for example, presence of physical/psychiatric causes, modification of environmental factors if any and reduction of stimuli/reinforcers of challenging behaviour.

Immediate management

- If the patient has evidence of mental *illness* and the risks are high then consider admission to a learning disability unit, possibility under the Mental Health Act (or a secure unit if there are serious risks involved).
- If the disturbed behaviour results from a psychiatric disorder, the treatment is similar in most ways to that for a patient of normal intelligence with the same disorder and in addition will also require a *behavioural regimen.*
- For agitated behaviour, try rapid tranquillization (first try oral medications and then parenteral injections).
- Discuss with the nursing team/manager and decide on level of nursing observation.
- If the behaviour is due to a physical cause, liaise with other specialties and their GP and treat it accordingly.

Other approaches

- Education – for both families/carers to improve understanding
- Impairments of vision, hearing and language – address these using sign language, use of pictures etc.
- Social interventions – address the unmet needs at home with family/carers and widen access to other services to improve support network

- Physical intervention – this varies from the use of splints, headgear and physical restraint to isolation in order to protect individual and others from injury or damage to property
- Behavioural therapy (see below).

Behavioural therapy

FUNCTIONAL BEHAVIOURAL ASSESSMENT – ABC CHART

This is based on accounts by family and carers and asks the parents or care staff to keep records of behaviour, such as eating, sleeping and general activity, so that problems can be identified and quantified.

'Record keeping' is an effective way of *defining the problem*, identifying relevant antecedents and consequences and informing management. A *diary* is a useful way of recording the information, identifying the problem, identifying the possible causes and establishing a baseline.

Institute the ABC analysis (antecedents, behaviour and consequences):

- Can *antecedents* (triggers) be identified?
- If so, can they be *modified* in order to prevent the challenging behaviour?
- Can *consequences* that reinforce the behaviour be identified? If so, can they be modified?

Role of CBT in the management of the learning-disabled population

- CBT is helpful for patients with high verbal ability and understanding if there is evidence of mood and/or anxiety disorders. (Mild LDs may be involved more in psychological than the moderate and the severe ones.)
- It may be effective in the management of anxiety and depressive disorders, the teaching of problem solving skills, dealing with issues of self-esteem and anger management. Use of CBT techniques, such as thought stopping, covert sensitization and aversive conditioning, may be helpful.

Pharmacotherapy

- The patients with LDs commonly experience *side effects,* particularly with the use of neuroleptics and both children and adults with LDs should be monitored closely if medication is to be prescribed.
- Antipsychotics are used for the treatment of co-morbid psychiatric disorders (schizophrenia and related psychosis) and acute behavioural disturbance.
- For episodes of serious aggression or agitation a trial of antipsychotic treatment may be useful. There is most experience with risperidone. Low-dose antipsychotics may reduce stereotypies.
- The other options for aggression, agitation and self-injurious behaviour include the use of anticonvulsants.

- Antidepressants, especially SSRIs, are mainly used for the treatment of depression, OCD and other anxiety disorders. They are also used for the treatment of self-injurious behaviour and other compulsive behaviour.
- Lithium is also used for the treatment of bipolar disorder and augmentation of antidepressant therapy.
- Lithium is licensed for the control of aggressive behaviour or intentional self-harm and it is the only drug licensed for the treatment of self-injurious behaviour.
- For self-injurious behaviour alone, there is some evidence for the use of opioid antagonists such as naltrexone hydrochloride. It may decrease repetitive self-injurious behaviour acutely but it is less effective in the long term.
- For specific co-morbid conditions, use the following:
  - For epilepsy use anticonvulsants
  - For depression use SSRIs and other antidepressant treatment
  - For OCD use SSRIs and other antidepressants
  - For ADHD use psychostimulants such as methylphenidate hydrochloride
- There is an increased prevalence of epilepsy in children with LDs, which is estimated at 6% in those with mild disability, 30% in those with moderate disability and 50% in those with severe disability (Rutter et al, 1970).
- Medical treatment for those with epilepsy who also have LDs is, in principle, the same as for those without LDs. However, it is much more complicated as the patients with LDs may exhibit different types of seizures and need combination treatment with different anticonvulsants.

Levels of learning disability

IQ defines this:

- Mild LD: IQ 50–69
- Moderate LD: IQ 35–49
- Severe LD: IQ 20–34
- Profound LD: IQ <20.

12

Specialist populations

Drug prescribing for specialist populations

Psychotropic prescribing in pregnancy

It is absolutely important to discuss with the woman the absolute and relative risks associated with treating and not treating the mental disorder before making treatment decisions. Also, it is important to explain the background risks of fetal malformation for pregnant women without a mental disorder, which is between 2 and 4 in 100 in the general population.

Antipsychotics

Low-dose chlorpromazine, low-dose haloperidol, low-dose trifluoperazine hydrochloride, olanzapine, clozapine.

Risks to consider:

- Weight gain and gestational diabetes with olanzapine
- Raised prolactin levels with risperidone, amisulpride and sulpiride.

Antidepressants

Fluoxetine hydrochloride, tricyclic antidepressants, such as amitriptyline, imipramine, nortriptyline.

Risks to consider:

- Fetal heart defects with paroxetine in the first trimester
- Persistent pulmonary hypertension in the neonate with selective serotonin (5-hydroxytryptamine) reuptake inhibitors (SSRIs) taken after 20 weeks' gestation.

Anxiolytics and hypnotics

Benzodiazepines are best avoided, but for sedation promethazine is widely used.

Mood stabilizers

Better to avoid unless risks and consequences of relapse outweigh known risk of teratogenesis.

Lithium

- There is an increased risk of Ebstein's anomaly (1:1000) and fetal heart defects.
- However, relapse rates are quite high – 50% within 1–2 months on discontinuation – which would normally preclude discontinuation in pregnancy.
- Detailed ultrasound or fetal echocardiography is indicated at 16–18 weeks.
- Serum monitoring and dosage adjustment, particularly during the second and third trimesters, is needed; also, ensuring adequate hydration after delivery is important.

Sodium valproate and carbamazepine

- Sodium valproate and carbamazepine are associated with neural tube defects.
- Detailed ultrasonography should be carried out at 16–18 weeks.
- Maternal serum alpha protein levels should be measured at 16–18 weeks.
- Folic acid supplementation is recommended for women of childbearing age.
- Vitamin K should be given to mothers in the last month of pregnancy and to neonates at birth due to the risk of neonatal haemorrhage.

Psychotropic prescribing in lactation

- Antipsychotics – sulpiride, olanzapine
- Antidepressants – sertraline hydrochloride, paroxetine hydrochloride, imipramine, nortriptyline hydrochloride
- Mood stabilizers – to be avoided if possible; lithium should be avoided; carbamazepine and sodium valproate should be used cautiously, to be given as a single dose in slow-release form
- Anxiolytics and hypnotics – lorazepam, zolpidem tartrate.

Psychotropic prescribing for patients with renal impairment

No drug is clearly preferred to another. They should be used with caution in exceptional circumstances.

- Antipsychotics – low dose haloperidol (2–5 mg/day), low dose olanzapine (5 mg/day)

- Antidepressants – sertraline hydrochloride, citalopram
- Mood stabilizers – sodium valproate, carbamazepine, lamotrigine at lower doses
- Anxiolytics and hypnotics – lorazepam, zopiclone.

Psychotropic prescribing for patients with hepatic impairment

- Antipsychotics – low dose haloperidol (2–5 mg/day), sulpiride, amisulpride
- Antidepressants – imipramine (low dose), paroxetine hydrochloride, citalopram
- Mood stabilizers – lithium
- Anxiolytics and hypnotics – lorazepam, temazepam, oxazepam, zopiclone.

Psychotropic prescribing for patients with cardiovascular disease

Post-myocardial infarction patients:

- Antidepressants – SSRIs, such as fluoxetine hydrochloride, paroxetine hydrochloride, sertraline hydrochloride, and low-dose trazadone hydrochloride
- Antipsychotics – low-dose haloperidol, olanzapine
- Avoid phenothiazines, tricyclic antidepressants, beta-blockers and hypotensive agents, such as clozapine, risperidone, and high-dose venlafaxine hydrochloride.

Psychotropic prescribing for patients with epilepsy

- Antipsychotics – haloperidol, sulpiride, amisulpride, zuclopenthixol, risperidone, quetiapine fumarate
- Antidepressants – SSRIs
- Mood stabilizers – carbamazepine, sodium valproate, lamotrigine, therapeutic doses of lithium
- Anxiolytics and hypnotics – all benzodiazepines can be used, as they are anticonvulsant in nature.

Psychotropic prescribing for patients with post-stroke depression

- SSRIs
- Nortriptyline hydrochloride.

Monitoring

Recommended plasma levels for selected drugs are given in Table 9.2.

TABLE **9.2** Recommended plasma levels for selected drugs

Drug	Recommended plasma level
Nortriptyline hydrochloride	50–150 mg/L
Amitriptyline	100–200 mg/L
Clozapine	350–500 mg/L
Olanzapine	20–40 mg/L
Lithium	0.8–1.2 mmol/L
Carbamazepine	4–12 mg/L
Sodium valproate	50–125 mg/L
Phenytoin	10–20 mg/L

Other medications commonly used in psychiatric practice

Anticholinergic medication

Side effects – dryness of the mouth, constipation, urinary hesitancy, blurred vision, dilation of the pupils, tachycardia, dizziness, euphoria, hallucinations, and delirium.

Recommended doses are given in Table 9.3.

TABLE **9.3** Recommended doses for anti-cholinergic drugs

Drug name	Usual recommended dosage (mg/day)
Procyclidine hydrochloride	2.5–30
Orphenadrine	150–400
Benzatropine mesilate	0.5–6
Benzhexol hydrochloride	2–15

Benzodiazepines

Side effects – drowsiness, dizziness, ataxia, respiratory depression, disinhibition in the elderly.

Recommended doses are given in Table 9.4.

Non-benzodiazepine alternatives

Side effects:

- Zopiclone – bitter taste, sedation, dry mouth, headaches, fatigue
- Zolpidem tartrate – headache, dizziness, drowsiness, gastrointestinal upsets

TABLE **9.4** Recommended doses for benzodiazepines

Drug name	Recommended dosages (mg/day)
Lorazepam	1–4
Temazepam	10–20
Nitrazepam	5–10
Oxazepam	15–90
Diazepam	2–30
Chlordiazepoxide	10–100
Alprazolam	0.25–1.5

- Buspirone hydrochloride – headaches, drowsiness, dizziness, nausea.

Recommended doses are given in Table 9.5.

TABLE **9.5** Recommended doses for non-benzodiazepine alternatives

Drug name	Recommended dosages (mg/day)
Zopiclone	7.5–1.5
Zolpidem tartrate	5–10
Buspirone hydrochloride	10–45

Drugs list

alprazolam	isocarboxazid
amisulpride	isoniazid
amoxapine	lamotrigine
aripiprazole	levodopa
atenolol	lorazepam
atomoxetine	methyldopa
biperiden	mirtazapine
buprenorphine	moclobemide
carbamazepine	nitrazepam
chlordiazepoxide	olanzapine
chlorpromazine	orlistat
cimetidine	orphenadrine
citalopram	oxazepam
clomipramine	phenytoin
clonazepam	pimozide
clozapine	pindolol
desipramine	pregabalin
dexamethasone	promethazine
dexamfetamine sulfate	reboxetine
diazepam	reserpine
disulfiram (Antabuse)	risperidone
escitalopram	rivastigmine
flupentixol decanoate	sibutramine
fluphenazine decanoate	sodium valproate
gabapentin	sulpiride
glycine	temazepam
haloperidol	topiramate
haloperidol decanoate	trimipramine
ibuprofen	tryptophan
imipramine	ziprasidone

zopiclone
zotepine
zuclopenthixol

zuclopenthixol acetate
zuclopenthixol decanoate

Drug name changes to rINN

acamprosate	acamprosate calcium
amitryptyline	amitriptyline
D-amphetamine	amphetamine
benzhexol	benzhexol hydrochloride
benztrophine	benzatropine mesilate
bromocriptine	bromocriptine mesilate
buspirone	buspirone hydrochloride
clonidine	clonidine hydrochloride
D-cycloserine	cycloserine
cyclosporine	ciclosporin
cyproheptadine	cyproheptadine hydrochloride
donepezil	donepezil hydrochloride
L-dopa	levodopa
dothiepin	dothiepin hydrochloride
doxepin	doxepin hydrochloride
duloxetine	duloxetine hydrochloride
fluoxetine	fluoxetine hydrochloride
flupenthixol	flupenthixol decanoate
fluvoxamine	fluvoxamine malate
galantamine	galantamine hydrobromide
levothyroxine	thyroxine sodium
lofepramine	lofepramine hydrochloride
Lofexidine	Lofexidine hydrochloride
loperamide	loperamide hydrochloride
maprotiline	maprotiline hydrochloride
memantine	memantine hydrochloride
methadone	methadone hydrochloride
methyl phenidate	methyl phenidate hydrochloride
metoclopramide	metoclopramide hydrochloride
mianserin	mianserin hydrochloride
naltrexone	naltrexone hydrochloride
nefazodone	nefazodone hydrochloride
nortryptyline	nortriptyline hydrochloride
paroxetine	paroxetine hydrochloride
phenelzine	phenelzine sulfate

pipothiazine decanoate   pipotiazine decanoate
procyclidine   procyclidine hydrochloride
propranolol   propranolol hydrochloride
quetiapine   quetiapine fumarate
sertraline   sertraline hydrochloride
sildenafil   sildenafil citrate
tranylcypromine   tranylcypromine sulfate
trazodone   trazodone hydrochloride
trifluoperazine   trifluoperazine hydrochloride
trihexyphenidyl   trihexyphenidyl hydrochloride
triiodothyronine   liothyronine sodium
venlafaxine   venlafaxine hydrochloride
vincristine   vincristine sulfate
yohimbine   yohimbine hydrochloride
zolpidem   zolpidem tartrate

References and further reading

References

Barbui C, Campomori A, D'Avanzo B, Negri E, Garattini S. (1999) Antidepressant drug use in Italy since the introduction of SSRIs: national trends, regional differences and impact on suicide rates. *Soc Psychiatry Psychiatr Epidemiol* **34**:152–6.

Barnard L, Young AH, Pearson J, Geddes J and O'Brian G. (2002) A systematic review of the use of atypical antipsychotics in autism. *J Psychopharmacol* **16**:93–101.

Chick J, Ritson B, Connaughton J, Stewart A, Chick J. (1988) Advice versus extended treatment for alcoholism: a controlled study. *Br J Addict* **83**:159–70.

Edwards G, Gross MM. (1976) Alcohol dependence: provisional description of a clinical syndrome. *Br Med J* **1**:1058–61.

Edwards G, Guthrie S. (1967) A controlled trial of inpatient and outpatient treatment of alcohol dependency. *Lancet* **1**:555–9.

Fairburn CG. (2005) Evidence-based treatment of anorexia nervosa. *Int J Eat Disord* **37** Suppl:S26–30; discussion S41–2.

Gabbard GO, Coyne L, Allen JG, Spohn H, Colson DB, Vary M. (2000) Evaluation of intensive inpatient treatment of patients with severe personality disorders. *Psychiatr Serv* **51**:893–8.

Koenig HG, George LK, Peterson BL, Pieper CF. (1997) Depression in medically ill hospitalized older adults: prevalence, characteristics, and course of symptoms according to six diagnostic schemes. *Am J Psychiatry* **154**:1376–83.

Lieberman JA, Koreen AR, Chakos M et al. (1996) Factors influencing treatment response and outcome of first-episode schizophrenia: implications for understanding the pathophysiology of schizophrenia. *J Clin Psychiatry* **57** Suppl 9:5–9.

McGrath J, Saha S, Welham J, El Saadi O, MacCauley C, Chant D. (2004) A systematic review of the incidence of schizophrenia: the distribution of rates and the influence of sex, urbanicity, migrant status and methodology. *BMC Med* **2**:13.

Miller WR, Hester RK. (1986) Inpatient alcoholism treatment. Who benefits? *Am Psychol* **41**:794–805.

Pane FJ, Ringer L, Ferguson L, Koshko N. (1991) Notifying patients of adverse drug reactions. *Am J Hosp Pharm* **48**:236–7.

Robinson DG, Woerner MG, Alvir JM et al. (1999) Predictors of treatment response from a first episode of schizophrenia or schizoaffective disorder. *Am J Psychiatry* **156**:544–9.

Russell GF, Szmukler GI, Dare C, Eisler I. (1987) An evaluation of family therapy in anorexia nervosa and bulimia nervosa. *Arch Gen Psychiatry* **44**:1047–56.

Rutter ML. (1970) Psycho-social disorders in childhood, and their outcome in adult life. *J R Coll Physicians Lond*. **4**:211–8.

Scott AI and Lock T. (1995) Monitoring seizure activity In *The ECT Handbook, 1E* (Ed. CP Freeman). pp. 62–66. Royal College of Psychiatrists, London.

Semple D, Smyth R, Burns J, Darjee R, McIntosh A. (2005) *Oxford Handbook of Psychiatry*. OUP, Oxford.

Tew JD Jr, Mulsant BH, Haskett RF et al. (1999) Acute efficacy of ECT in the treatment of major depression in the old. *Am J Psychiatry* **156**:1865–70.

Further reading

Ahuja N. (2001) *A Short Texbook of Psychiatry*. 4E, Jaypee Brothers Medical Publishers Ltd., London.

Andrews G, Jenkins R. (1999) *Management of Mental Disorders* 2E. WHO Collaborating Centers for Mental Health and Substance Abuse. Geneva.

Bhugra D, Malik A and Brown N. (2007) *Workplace Based Assessments in Psychiatry*. RCPsych publications. http://www.rcpsych.ac.uk

British National Formulary, (2008) BMJ Publishing, London.

Gelder M, Cowen P, Harrison P. (2006) 5E *Shorter Oxford Textbook of Psychiatry*, OUP, Oxford.

Goodwin G, Sachs G. (2004) *Bipolar Affective Disorder*. Icon Group International.

ICD-10 Classification of Mental Behavioral Disorders, Clinical Descriptions and Diagnostic Guidelines 2E. (2002) AITBS Publishers and Distributors.

Kane JM. (2000) *Management Issues in Schizophrenia*. 1E, Martin Dunitz, Abington.

Lewis SW, Buchanan RW. (2002) *Schizophrenia*: *Fast Facts in Psychiatry*. 2E. Fine Print Services Ltd. Oxford.

Murthy SPM (2008) *Get Through MRCPsych: Preparation for the CASC*. RSM Press, London.

Semple D, Smyth R, Burns J, Darjee R, McIntosh A. (2005) *Oxford Handbook of Psychiatry*. OUP, Oxford.

Taylor D, Paton C, Kerwin R.(2005–06) *The Maudsley Prescribing Guidelines, 8E*. Taylor & Francis, London.

Wolff K, Farrell M, Marsden J, Monteiro MG, Ali R, Welch S, Strang J. (1999) A review of biological indicators of illicit drug use, practical considerations and clinical usefulness. *Addiction* **94**:1279–98.

Williams C, Trigwell P, Yeomans D. (2002) *Pass the MRCPsych Part 1 and 2 2E*. WB Saunders, London.

Guidelines

NICE guidelines: Advances in psychiatric treatment Jan 2004–Jan 2006 www.nice.org.uk

American Psychiatric Association, 2002. http://www.psych.org